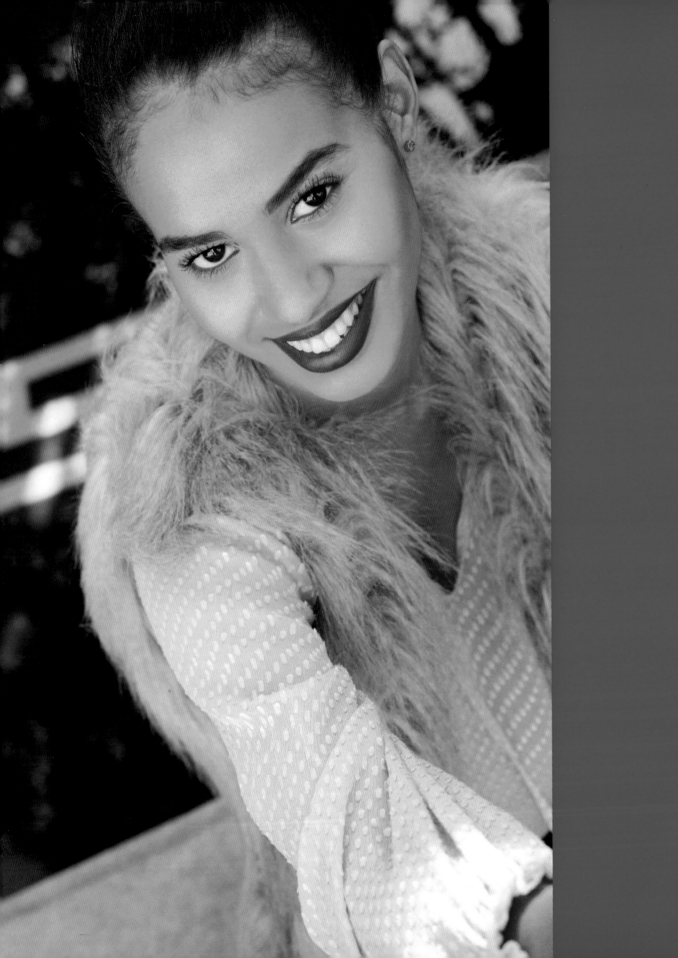

#beautiful

by Luis Casco

5o

Easy-to-create
selfie-ready
beauty looks

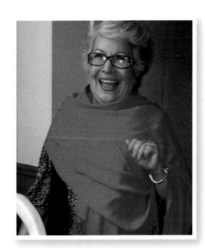

I dedicate this book to my mom.
Without her support, encouragement and love, this project wouldn't have been possible.

Love, Luis

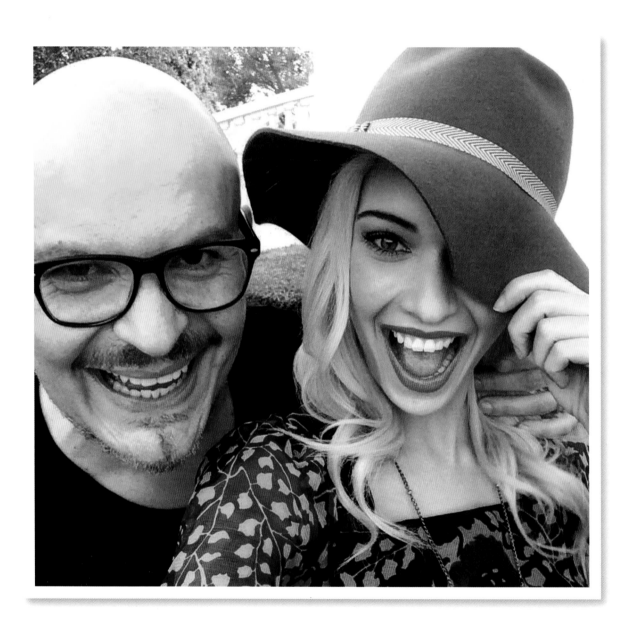

In an incredibly short period of time, the word "selfie" has become ubiquitous around the world. Of course, there have always been self-portraits — artists and amateurs alike have drawn, painted and photographed their likeness for art and posterity throughout history. But never before has the ability to create hundreds of versions at one time, instantly visible and at virtually no cost, been possible. Now every teenager, mother and grandmother has the ability to hold out her phone and snap a selfie. Not to mention the luxury of looking at it instantly (ask your grandmother how long she used to have to wait to see her snapshots), deciding it might look better with her chin down and taking a dozen more shots until she gets it just right.

Twitter declared 2014 as "The Year of the Selfie," but I'd bet money there will be more selfies taken in 2015 than ever before. We use them to share moments with our friends, family and followers. We use them as our profile pictures on social media. I even saw a printed selfie Christmas card last year! The selfie gives us total control — we can take as many as we need until we get the perfect shot. I would bet there are tens of thousands of people who have a favorite selfie that they believe is the best picture anyone has ever taken of them.

The selfie craze has had a major impact on my life and career, as well. For years I've worked with celebrities, models, photographers and crews and made fast friendships, but because of the nature of our work, I often wouldn't see them again for many years. Even though I would hold onto professional images from editorial or advertising jobs, I didn't usually take or keep candid shots of the shoot. Now, I document everything with my smartphone and I take a selfie with virtually every model on set. And in case you were wondering, models know how to take excellent selfies! I just hand the phone to them and say, "Take a selfie of us." They know their angles, they know how to crop and they aren't afraid to take a couple dozen shots before they hand the phone back to me. These selfies are a great way to document my work, because I'm the one who did the model's makeup!

My idea for this book grew out of those experiences. When you know your angles and you know how to crop — and you are wearing amazing makeup — you can take truly spectacular selfies.

In this book, I share easy-to-create makeup tips and I challenge you to think about your location, your surroundings, what you want in your selfie and what you don't. I give you tips on lighting and suggestions for the best angles for your face.

To produce the book, I held a casting in Los Angeles with models, actresses and "normal" women. I selected 25+ women of various ages and with a variety of skin tones. I partnered with my friend, the very talented photographer Peter Augustin, and over a period of seven days, we shot all of the images in this book. It was at times exhausting but also very rewarding to see the project come to life.

Peter took the beautiful before-and-after shots to illustrate what we did to each model, but all of the finished selfie looks are real selfies. Each image was taken by the model with a smartphone. I point this out just to emphasize that all of these looks and shots are attainable.

Are you using a picture of your cat as your profile picture? Or a shot of a sunset from your last vacation because you don't have any pictures of yourself that you think are "good enough?" If so, I hope you'll take some inspiration from this book and realize that you, too, can take a great selfie.

So tag me **@luiscascomakeup** — I'd love to see what you do with some (or all!) of the 50 looks I created for this book! ☺

TABLE OF CONTENTS

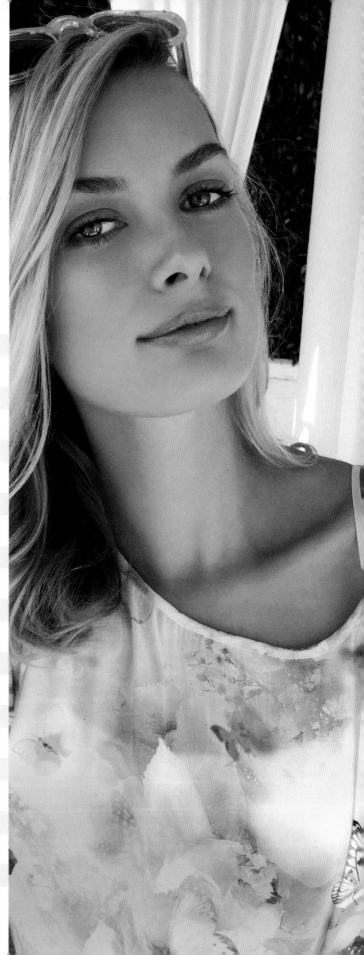

The Looks:

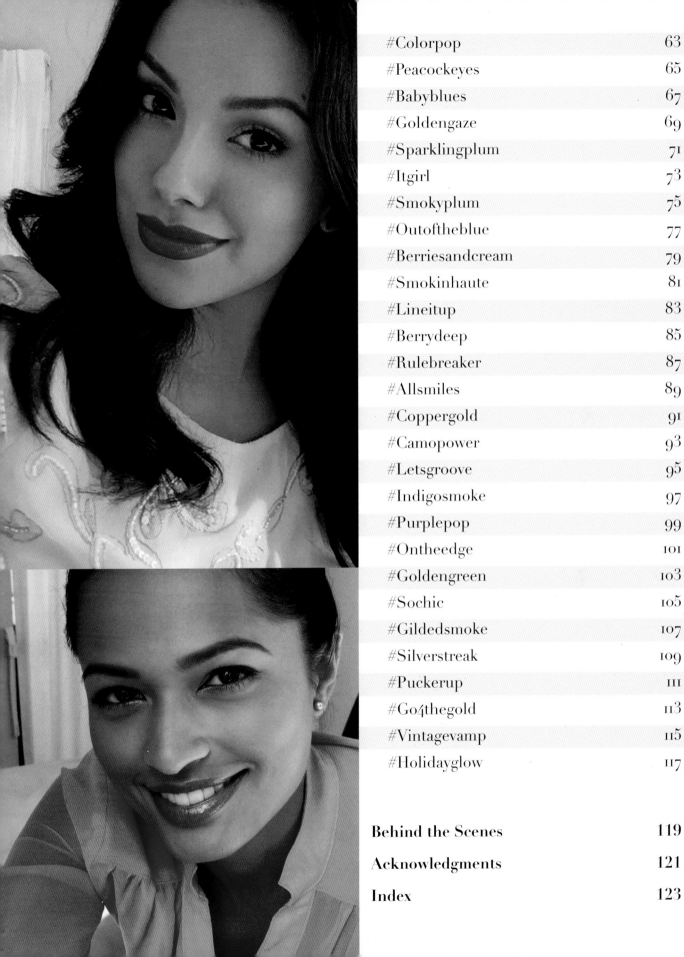

THE ANATOMY OF AN AWESOME SELFIE

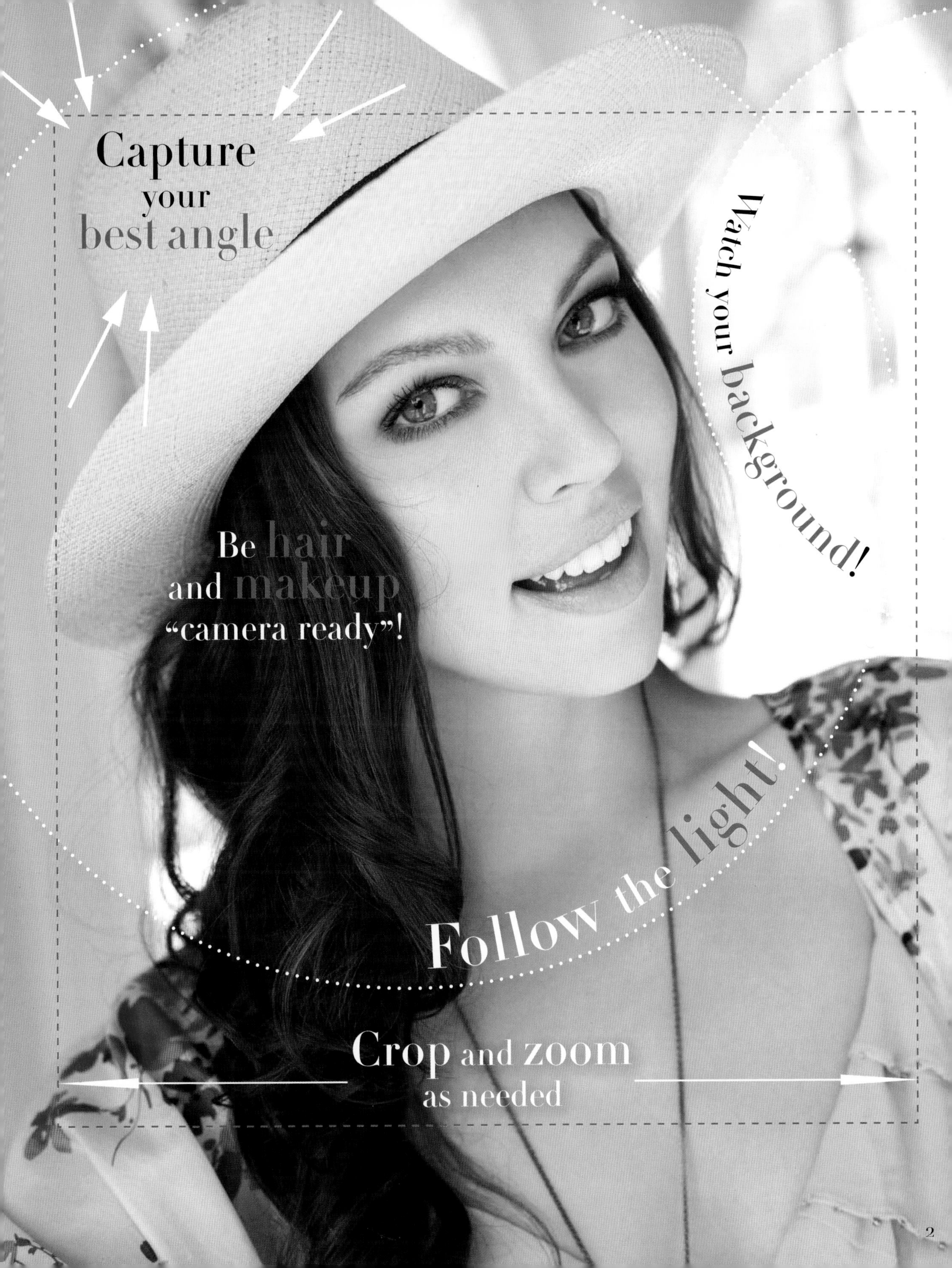

Capture
your
best angle

Watch your background!

Be hair
and makeup
"camera ready"!

Follow the light!

Crop and zoom
as needed

HOW TO
take the BEST
SELFIES

The world has gone selfie crazy!

A study called #selfiegraphic by Techinfographics.com gives us some staggering figures. There are one million selfies taken each day and of those, 36% of people admit to digitally altering them.

Selfies are being shared the most on:

Facebook 48%

WhatsApp Messenger and Text 27%

Twitter 9%

Instagram 8%

Snapchat 5%

Pinterest 2%

Clearly, Selfies are here to stay! So here are 26 dos and don'ts to ensure you always get a great shot.

Selfie DOs

1. **Know your best angles.** Knowing your angles can make or break your selfie. But this doesn't just mean knowing which side of your face you like better. It's also about the angle at which you hold your smartphone. Low angles tend to create double chins — and no one needs that. Holding your smartphone at eye level or slightly above, with your face looking straight into the camera, makes you look the most natural. A selfie taken from a higher angle typically has more shadows and highlights, which can make your face appear slimmer and your eyes appear slightly larger. Once you've figured out the best camera angle, you can give more thought to the way you angle your face and body. For instance, look at the model in the picture below. She's holding her face at a 3/4 angle, tilted slightly toward camera.

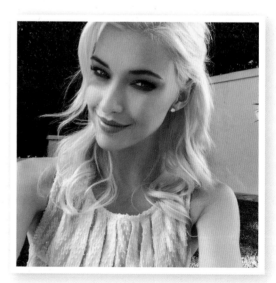

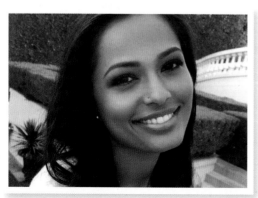

2. **Explore both the front and back-facing cameras.** If you have a smartphone that has both a front and back-facing camera, keep in mind that the two lenses are not usually of equal quality. Normally, the lens that is on the back of the smartphone is a more finely crafted lens. The picture quality will be higher when taken with that lens. The lens on the screen-side of the smartphone is easier to use for selfies — and it's the one I favor using personally — but the picture quality is not as good. In this book, both the front and back-facing lenses were used. See if you can tell which is which.

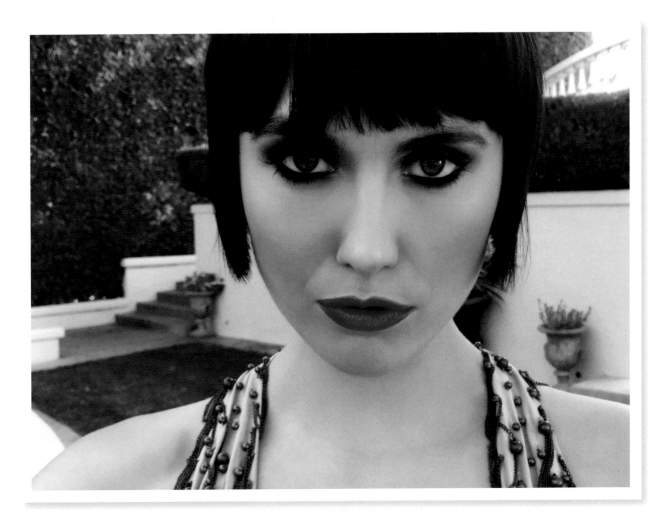

3. **Think about where you're looking.** Think about the mood and impression you want to communicate with your selfie. If you look straight into the lens of the camera, you create eye contact with the person looking at the shot. This is the classic way to take a selfie and the one I prefer. But looking away from the lens can give the shot an added layer of interpretation, even drama. And if you're taking a selfie with someone else — your best friend, for example — you may want to look at them. It's a cool way to add another level of meaning to your selfie.

4. **Get a selfie stick.** Want to see a little more of your look or take a selfie with a few friends in the frame? A selfie stick allows the positioning of a smartphone or camera to extend beyond the normal range of the arm, giving you the chance to show off even more in your selfies!

5. **Have something to say!** Selfies are a great tool for sharing bits about your life with the world. People want to see your new lipstick color or what makeup you're wearing to an event, so use this to your advantage and show off.

6. **Always add #hashtags.** Adding hashtags like #selfie, #beautiful, and #makeup to your descriptions is not only a great way to show up on other people's feeds, but is also a cool way of organizing your posts.

7. **Look your best.** Obviously, you want to look your best in your selfie. Make sure you moisturize your skin and lips to avoid any flakiness that might show. And capture yourself in the best possible way.

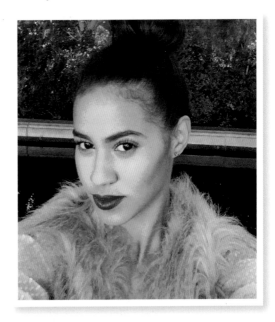

8. SMILE. When in doubt, a smile can serve as your best accessory. It engages the viewers and its effect can be contagious.

9. Let your personality shine through. Show the viewer who you are!

10. Filter away. Use filters to your advantage. They can really enhance your appearance when used smartly. Filters can make your skin look super smooth and enhance your makeup looks, as well. Brightening up and adding a fun effect to your picture can create a great selfie. Just remember that it's easy to over do it. If you use a filter that's over-the-top and tweaked, it may look more like an art project and less like a #beautiful selfie. So choose wisely. Filters and photo apps are easy to download and are often free.

11. Crop. Cropping can really change a picture and make it look cleaner and more compelling. Don't be afraid to zoom in or crop when necessary.

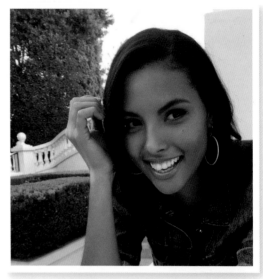

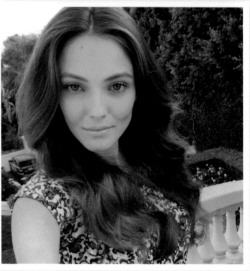

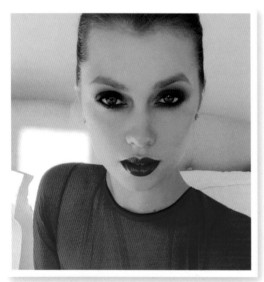

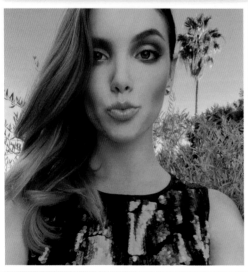

12. Choose your backgrounds wisely. Remember that the more you want to stand out in the picture, the more neutral the background should be.

13. Light it well. Always make an effort to find the best lighting. Natural, diffused light from a window or outdoors is the best. But harsh, direct overhead sunlight can cast unflattering shadows on your face, so be careful. Look for a spot that is bright but shielded, like underneath an awning or in the shadow of a building. Indoor light and mood lighting can also work well. Just be aware that some light bulbs give off either warmish yellow or cold blue light. I wouldn't recommend them for showing off great makeup.

14. To flash or not to flash? I rarely use a flash for selfies. Even in the dark light of a restaurant or outside at night, a flash tends to make selfies look garish. Most photo apps give you the ability to brighten and lighten pictures. Of course, there are times when you have to use a flash. But even so, it's still a good idea to use a photo app and adjust levels to make the shot look perfect.

Selfie DON'Ts

15. Don't overdo the makeup. Stick to one main feature to highlight and keep the rest of the face neutral. For instance, a bold lip will look great with a neutral, soft eye. Of course, you can be yourself and overdo it if that's what you like, but for most people this will make it look like they're trying too hard.

16. Don't forget about your hair! It's all about creating a pretty picture, so even if you haven't had time to do your hair, flipping it over once and then flipping it to one side can make your mane look amazing.

17. Don't Ignore your background. Remember to keep things simple and crop out anything behind you that you don't want people to see or associate with you.

18. Don't fall victim to the trends. Overly drawn out "Instagram brows" or heavily contoured skin are two examples of this. Keep your look fresh and natural unless you are trying to make a major statement.

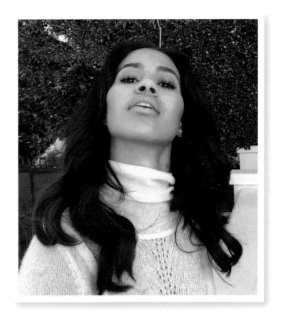

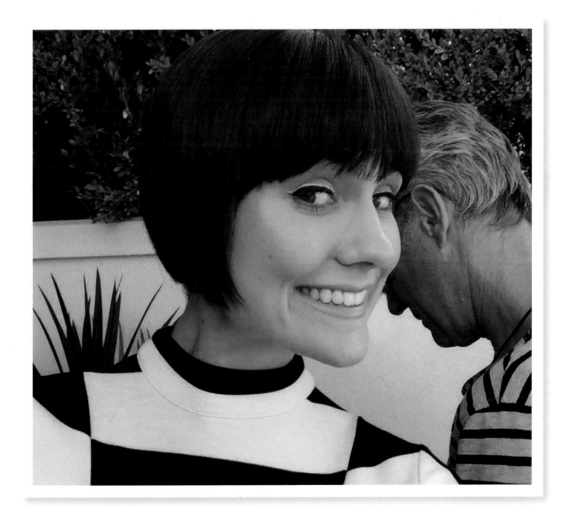

19. Don't forget to use concealer. Dark circles can make you look tired and older than you are. Use a concealer that's at least one shade lighter than your skin tone to brighten up the area under your eyes.

20. Don't ignore your lashes. They really make your eyes stand out and can look especially amazing in selfies. Even if you don't have a lot of time, one quick coat of mascara will always do the trick!

21. Don't be afraid to take tons of options of one look. This is something I've learned from years of experience. It's better to have plenty of options to choose from, so shoot away!

22. Don't share things that are too personal. T.M.I. is never a good thing. Remember that this picture of you is going out for all the world to see.

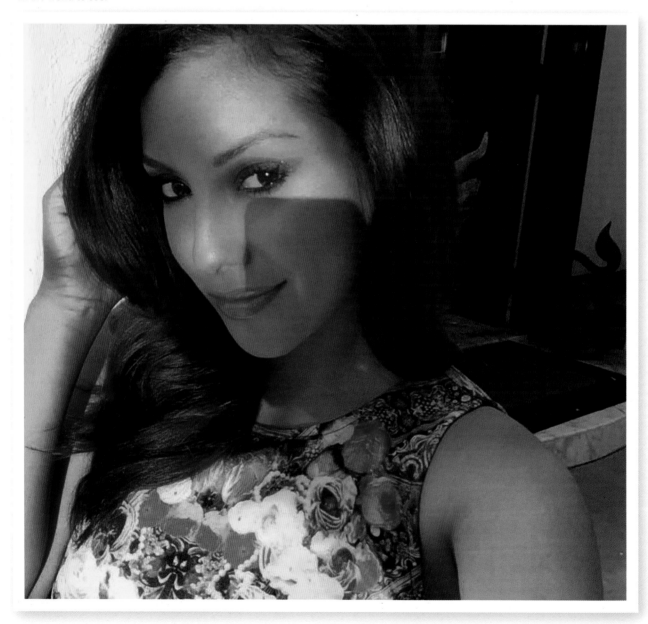

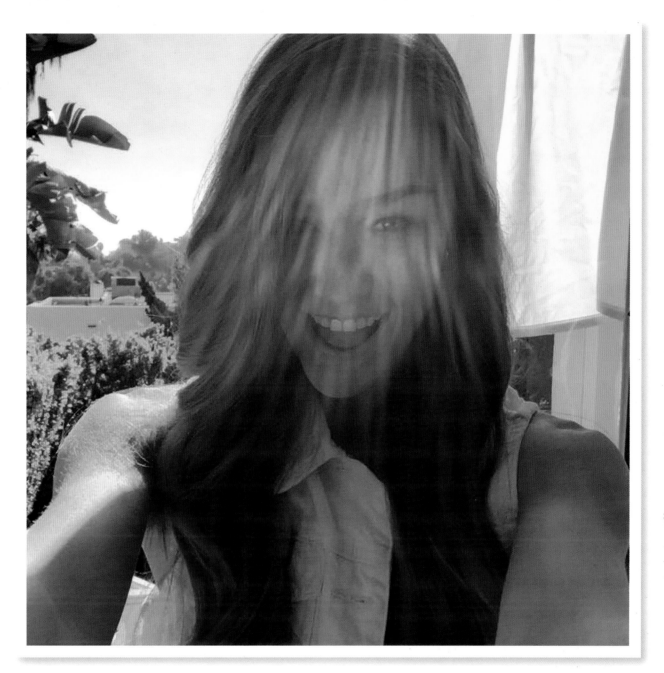

23. **Don't use too many hashtags.** A few compelling ones are all you need. Remember these words are automatically associated with you so, it's important not to take them lightly!

24. **Don't ignore the lighting.** Taking a selfie in a mirror with overhead lighting, for instance, will give you lots of unwanted dark circles and spots. Keep the light in front of you, instead.

25. **Don't take all your selfies in the same direction.** Some people's faces photograph better in a horizontal (landscape) composition, while others look better in a vertical shot. Experiment, have fun, and see what works best for you.

26. **Don't forget to tag me on your #selfies! @luiscascomakeup**

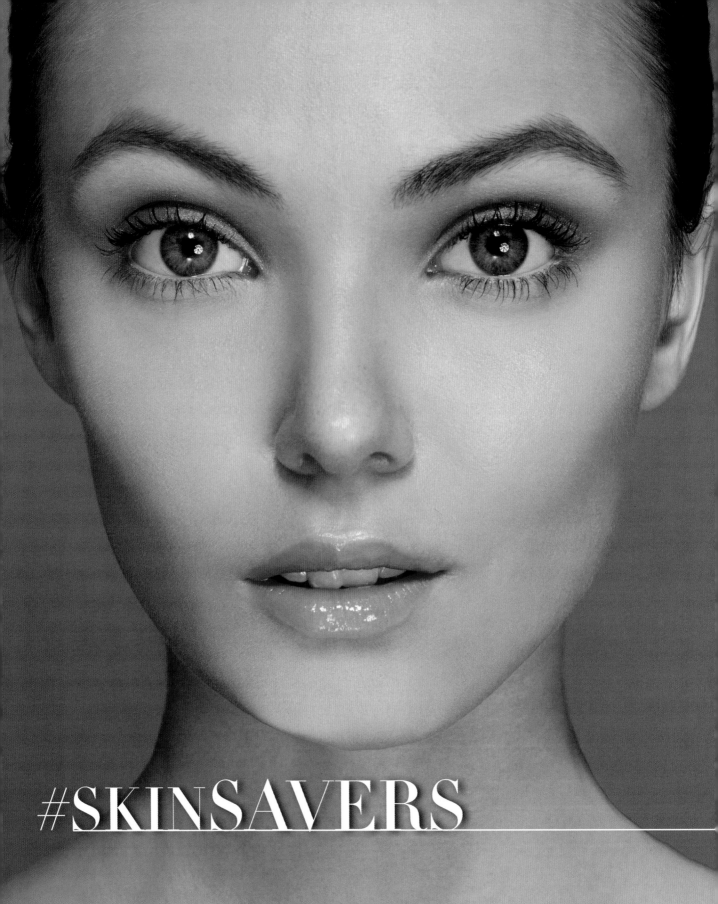

#SKINSAVERS

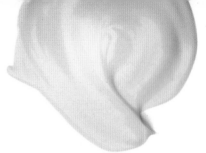

The way your skin looks in a picture can say so much about you.
That's why, as a makeup artist, I'm obsessed with helping people achieve the look of perfect skin. Here are some of my favorite tricks to help you create a beautiful canvas for your selfies. I am not an esthetician, so most of these are quick fixes, but they're great shortcuts for making your skin look flawless.

When it comes to great skin, you are either born with it, have to work to maintain it, or can do a really great job at faking it. I will concentrate on the last two options here!

Clean It!

This is a pretty basic tip, but washing your face twice a day is important — even more so if you wear makeup. At the very least, you need to make sure you take your makeup off each evening and cleanse your skin properly.

Look for a cleanser with ingredients like fatty acids, which help lock in moisture and have anti-inflammatory benefits. Make sure you find hypoallergenic formulas that are also non-comedogenic (which means they won't clog pores).

Another tool I highly recommend using is a face cleansing brush. It can really change the look of your skin. Just make sure you don't overdo it and use it only about every other day, depending on your skin type. Face cleansing brushes not only deep clean but also help prep the skin so that any skin care product you apply after you cleanse (such as moisturizer) will absorb easily.

SELFIE TIP: *Use a face mask a couple of times a week to help exfoliate the skin. The morning of your shoot, apply a brightening mask to make your skin look radiant. This is something I encourage all my clients to do and I'll even use one on them if time allows.*

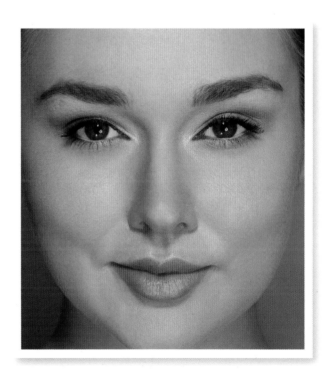

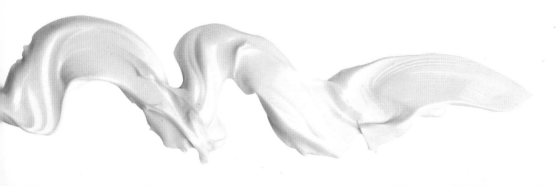

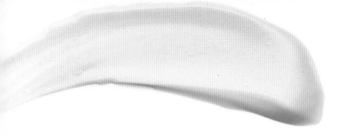

Hydrate It!

Dull, dehydrated skin is one of the worst things to have to deal with for a picture. Flaky, patchy skin can show up even when you're wearing makeup, so be sure to use a moisturizer no matter what type of skin you have.

Serums

I use serums on almost everyone. These potent potions deliver a high concentration of active ingredients that can immediately brighten dark spots, hydrate skin and create the ultimate prep for foundation. They're key if you wear makeup on a regular basis.

SELFIE TIP: *Try applying a serum on slightly damp, just-cleansed skin for maximum benefits.*

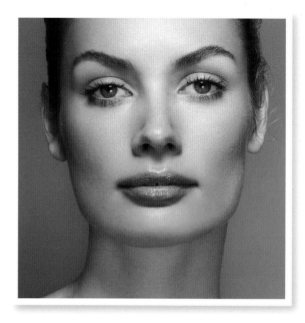

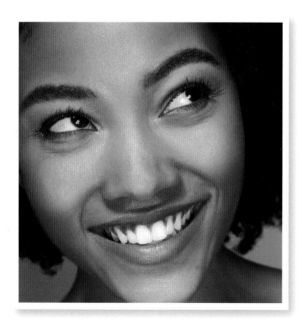

Eye Cream

It's a fact that the skin around your eyes is the thinnest and most sensitive, and it shows signs of aging the fastest. So if you are not using an eye cream yet — no matter what your age — start now! They will help minimize dark circles, wrinkles and puffiness.

SELFIE TIP: *Let a layer of eye cream "sit" under your eyes while you do the rest of your makeup. The hydrating and brightening benefits will help your concealer do a better job and you'll be able to see a big difference!*

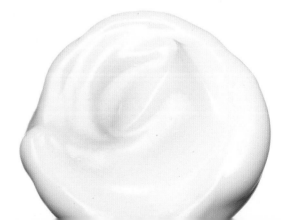

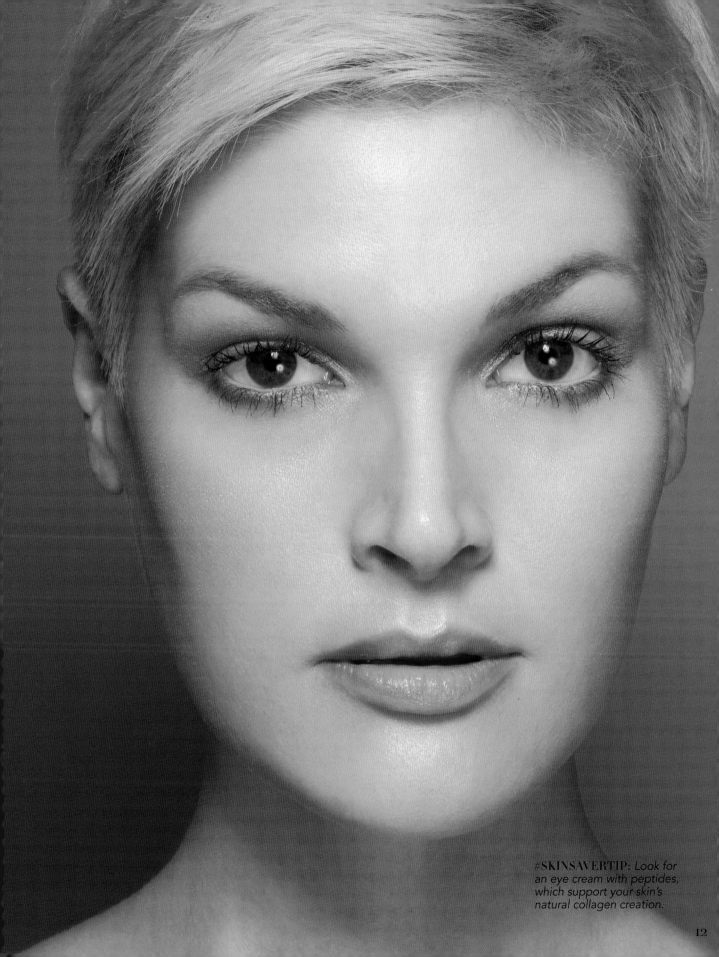

#SKINSAVERTIP: *Look for an eye cream with peptides, which support your skin's natural collagen creation.*

12

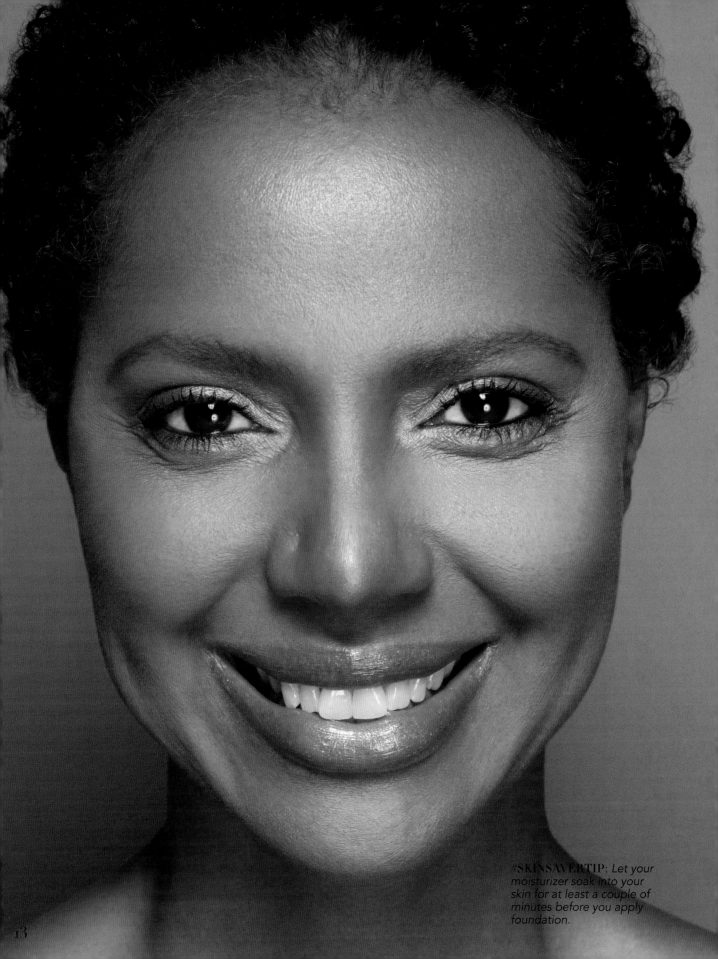

#SKINSAVERTIP: *Let your moisturizer soak into your skin for at least a couple of minutes before you apply foundation.*

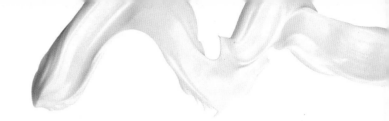

Moisturizer

Rub moisturizer in between your hands to activate the ingredients, then apply with firm circular motions — first to your cheeks, then to your forehead and nose and lastly on the chin and down the neck.

You should use both a daytime and nighttime formula of moisturizer. The daytime moisturizer should contain sunscreen to protect skin from the damage caused by sunlight and environmental exposure. The nighttime moisturizer should be designed to soothe and repair the skin while you sleep.

Sunscreen or foundation containing sunscreen can cause your skin to reflect a white cast, making the face look lighter than the rest of the body. Why? Sunscreen contains titanium dioxide and zinc oxide — two ingredients that tend to make faces look pale, especially in photographs. The best way to avoid this? Take a test selfie with a flash to make sure your face doesn't look wan or washed out.

SELFIE TIP: *As a firm believer in the importance of wearing sunscreen, one thing I've found to work well is to apply a layer of sunscreen to clean skin, let it absorb for about 10 minutes and then apply your foundation. Most of the time, this will give you the protection you need without adding that unwanted "white cast" to your skin.*

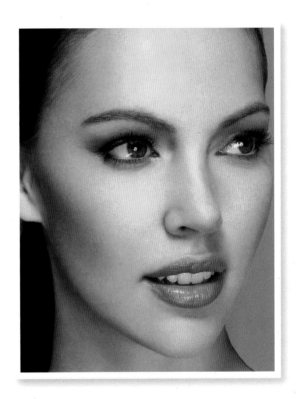

Face and Eyeshadow Primers

Primers can add major lasting power to your makeup and help hide a multitude of skin issues before you even apply foundation. Face primers come in silicon and silicon-free versions, so use the formula that works best for you. Eyeshadow primers add vibrancy and prevent creasing — I use them a lot when creating eye makeup looks.

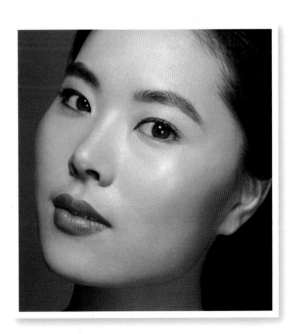

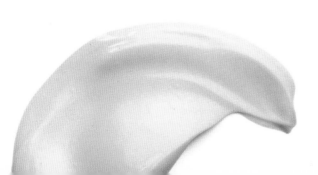

#SKINCAREPROTIPS

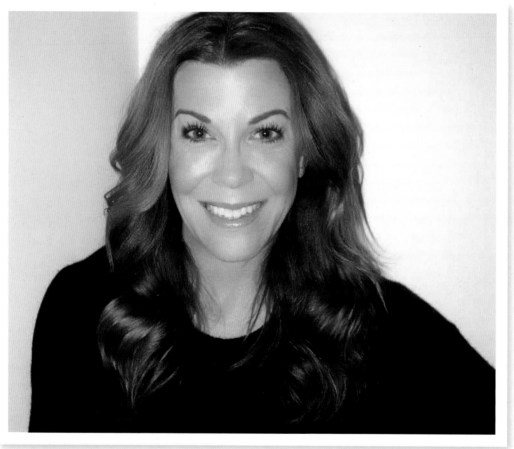

Carolyn Holdsworth, renowned esthetician and owner of Nurture Spa (www.nurturespa.com)

In order to give you some more tips from a professional, I contacted my friend Carolyn Holdsworth, renowned esthetician and owner of Nurture Spa (www.nurturespa. com), a luxury day spa in New Hope, Pennsylvania. She has a passion for skin care and is a seasoned beauty expert with years of experience.   Here are her top five skin care tricks.

My Top 5 Skincare Tips
for #BEAUTIFUL Skin

1. **Apply serums,** eye creams and facial moisturizers within three minutes of washing your face or leaving the shower. By applying products quickly after cleansing, you're helping to seal in hydration. This goes for your body as well — you should moisturize within three minutes of bathing. You'll enjoy longer-lasting, silky-smooth skin.

2. **Do not pick at blemishes!** The rule is, if it's not white, leave it alone. Picking at anything on your face will create more inflammation and redness and could possibly result in a scar. Instead of picking, apply a product with salicylic acid or benzoyl peroxide to the blemish and be patient. It will go away, I promise.

3. **Exfoliate your face daily,** with either chemical or manual exfoliants. In order for products to penetrate the epidermis and perform as they are intended, the dead skin cells must first be removed. A washcloth is a manual exfoliant, while vitamin C or vitamin A based products are wonderful chemical exfoliants. When you exfoliate regularly, your serums and moisturizers will be able to penetrate the skin more effectively, and your makeup will go on smoother and more evenly.

4. **Facial serums are worth the investment.** My favorite ingredient in a serum is hyaluronic acid, because it hydrates, smoothes and ignites collagen production, which can soften fine lines. A little goes a long way, so invest in the best product you can find, and use sparingly but daily. You'll see the difference instantly after application. If I'm on a budget, I will skimp on let's say, a cleanser, so I can invest in a high-quality serum that will deliver real results.

5. **Don't be afraid to be dewy!** The majority of my clients are afraid of oils and fear a shiny face, so they opt for oil-free products. Very few people need oil-free products, and you're actually creating a bigger problem if you intentionally dehydrate your skin. Allowing your skin to receive good-for-you oils and other hydrators will give you a fresh, youthful glow, and the shiny look will disappear before you know it. But if you can't wait for that little bit of shine to disappear, dust a small amount of translucent powder on your nose and chin. Just don't wipe off all the hydrating goodness!

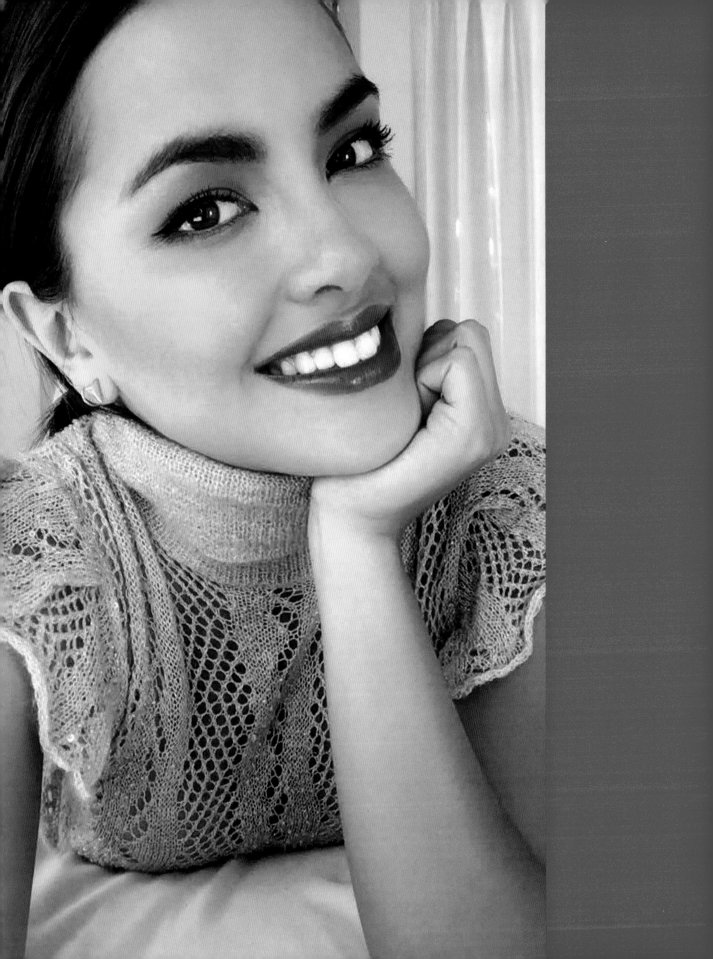

The 50
Looks

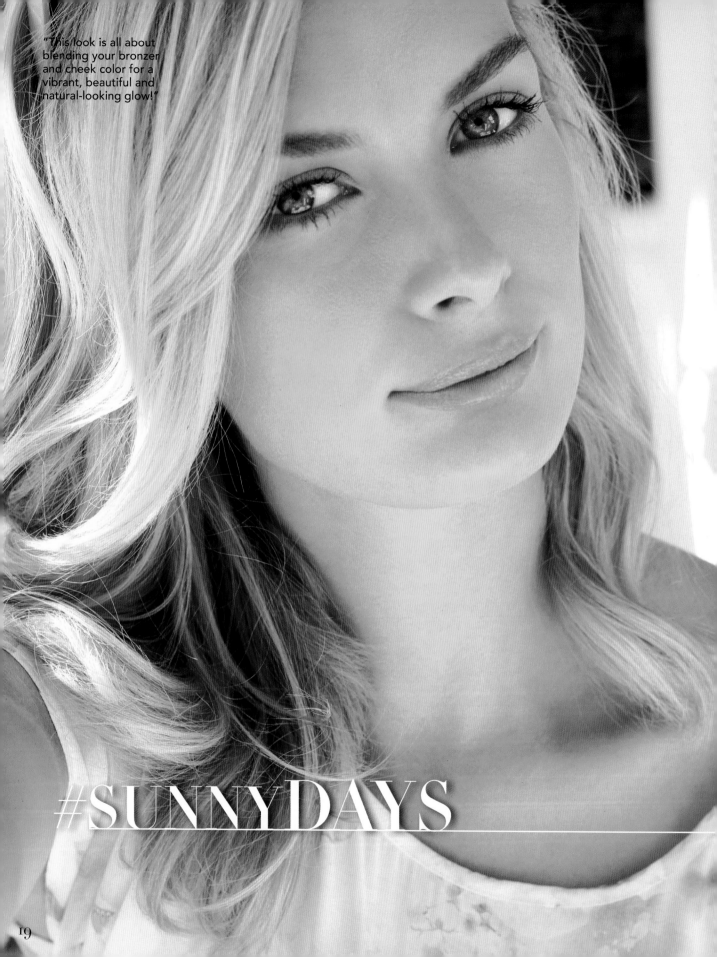

"This look is all about blending your bronzer and cheek color for a vibrant, beautiful and natural-looking glow!"

#SUNNYDAYS

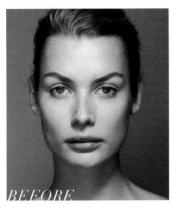

BEFORE

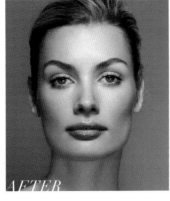

AFTER

The Essentials

- Light golden brown eyeshadow
- Volumizing mascara
- Concealer one shade lighter than your skin tone
- A peachy pink cheek color
- Bronzer
- An angled cheek brush
- Powder (or kabuki) brush, eyeshadow brush
- Peachy light brown lipstick or lip gloss

one

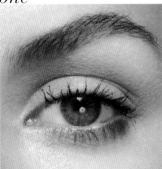

EYES: Apply eye primer to your eyelids and let dry. Using an eyeshadow brush, dust a shimmery light brown eyeshadow onto the base of your eyelids, starting at the inside corners and working outwards from lashline to just above the crease. Blend thoroughly with a clean crease brush to avoid any visible edges. Add concealer under your eyes, from the inner to outer corners along the lash line.

TIP: *If desired, add a tiny bit of concealer under your eyebrows to highlight your brow bone. Finish with a coat of volumizing mascara in black.*

SKIN: Prime your skin with moisturizer, then place a dot of BB or CC cream on the tip of your nose, forehead, cheeks and chin. Blend with your fingertips and dust a translucent powder over your T-zone.

CHEEKS: Smile in front of a mirror and dust a peachy pink blush onto the apples of your cheeks with a cheek brush. Use a clean cheek brush to sweep some bronzer onto the hollows of the cheeks and blend with the blush, making sure that all edges disappear at the hairline. Use any product left on the brush to bronze the highest peaks of the face (such as the hairline by the temples, the chin and the tip of the nose). Use another clean powder brush to soften any visible edges for the most natural, sun-kissed look. Add a nude sparkly gloss to finish the look!

two

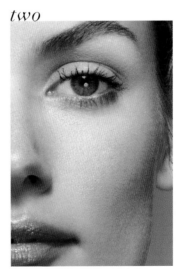

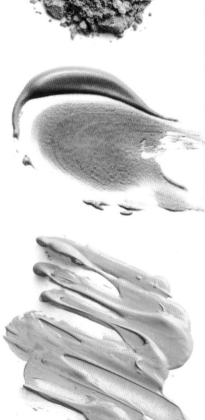

SELFIE TIP:
If your face has strong features, try photographing it from a few different angles — it pays to know how to take a selfie in the most flattering way!

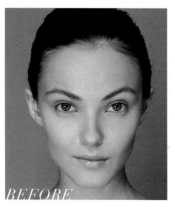

BEFORE

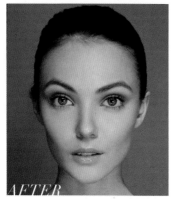

AFTER

The Essentials

- Foundation
- Foundation brush
- Translucent powder
- Bronzer
- Rosy blush
- Powder highlighter
- Cheek and powder brushes
- Sparkly nude lip gloss

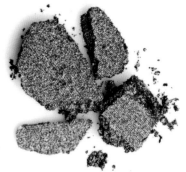

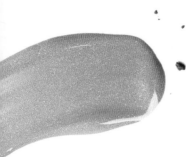

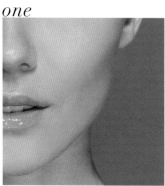

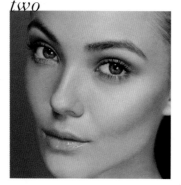

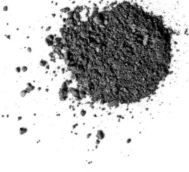

one

two

three

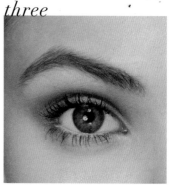

SKIN: Apply primer to cleansed and moisturized skin. Place a dot of foundation onto the center of the forehead, tip of the nose, cheeks and chin. Use a foundation brush to blend, concentrating on the areas where you need the most coverage. Blend until the foundation is undetectable, then follow with a very light layer of translucent loose powder.

TIP: *If you want to skip powder try using oil blotting sheets. They will absorb extra oils and leave your makeup intact!*

CHEEKS & LIPS: With a bronzer, sculpt the hollows of the cheeks, under the jawline and around the hairline. Dust your neck and décolletage with what's left on the brush so the color blends seamlessly with your skin. Apply a rosy hued blush onto the apples of your cheeks. Follow by blending a highlighter into the inner corners of the eyes, tops of the cheek bones, brow bone and Cupid's bow. Finish with a sparkly nude lip gloss.

EYES: Apply a golden bronze eye shadow or a bronzer to your lid from lash line to crease. Blend well and finish with two coats of mascara.

SELFIE TIP:

Try going outside when taking a selfie of this makeup look. Daylight automatically gives the skin a gorgeous glow!

#GLOWING

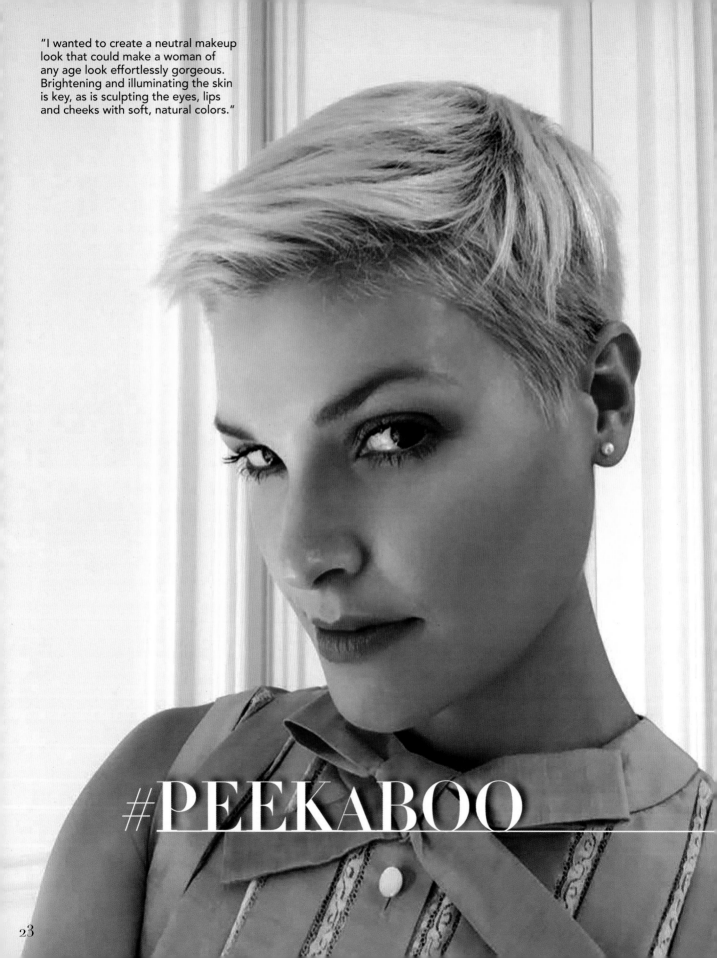

"I wanted to create a neutral makeup look that could make a woman of any age look effortlessly gorgeous. Brightening and illuminating the skin is key, as is sculpting the eyes, lips and cheeks with soft, natural colors."

#PEEKABOO

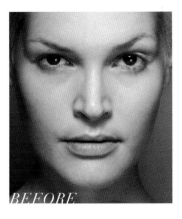

BEFORE

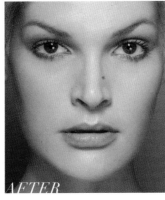

AFTER

The Essentials

- Luminous foundation, BB or CC cream
- Concealer
- Facial highlighter
- Shimmery taupe eyeshadow
- Mascara
- Eyeshadow and eyeliner brush
- Blush and lipstick in a shade that complements your skin tone (see below)

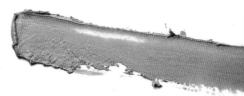

one

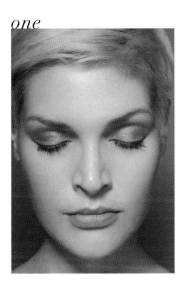

SKIN: Moisturize and add primer to skin. Apply a thin veil of foundation, starting from the center of the face and spreading outward. Dab concealer onto the outer and inner corners of the eye and around the edges of the nose. Blend well. Smooth a highlighter onto the upper portion of the cheeks, forehead, brow bone and inner corners of the eyes. Set with a light dusting of translucent powder over the T-zone.

TIP: *In a hurry? Use a BB or CC cream instead of foundation. They're all-in-one skin correctors that smooth imperfections and have immediate benefits, like sun protection and skin hydration.*

CHEEKS & LIPS: Here are some great blush and lipstick shade suggestions for different types of skin tones. They just might become your go-to hues!

   Fair: Light pink, coral, soft apricot

   Medium: Mauve, apricot, warm pink

   Dark: Dark brown, tangerine, cinnamon

two

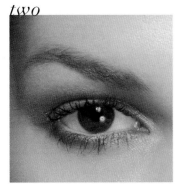

EYES: To emphasize your eyes in a natural-looking way, use an eyeshadow brush to apply a shimmery taupe eyeshadow over the lid, into the crease and along the bottom lash line. Press a charcoal or brown eyeshadow into the roots of the upper lashes with a stiff eyeliner brush.

TIP: *"Tightlining" the eyes by creating a thin, barely visible line right along the lashes makes your eyes look bigger and your lashes look thicker!*

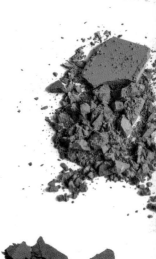

SELFIE TIP:

Posture is key! Slouching looks bad on camera and even shows in close-up shots. When taking a selfie, try to keep your back straight and shoulders up — it will make all the difference!

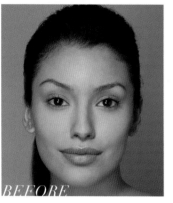

BEFORE

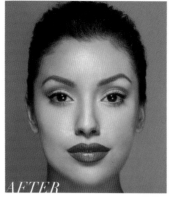

AFTER

The Essentials

- Foundation
- Translucent powder
- Eyeshadow in a color one shade lighter than your skin tone
- Light nude and matte brown eyeshadows
- Black gel or pencil eyeliner
- Mascara
- Warm rosy blush
- Golden chocolate lip liner
- Golden chocolate lipstick

one

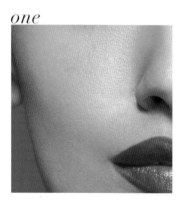

two

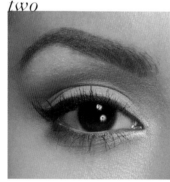

three

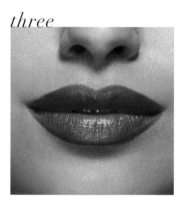

SKIN: Moisturize the skin and prime, if necessary. Dab a small amount of foundation onto your chin, forehead, nose and cheeks. Blend towards the outer edges of the face with your fingertips or a foundation brush. For a flawless yet natural-looking finish, use a damp sponge to blend out the foundation, making it as sheer as possible. Set with a light layer of powder.

EYES: Dust eyeshadow in a shade lighter than your skin tone onto your eyelids from the lashes to the brow bones. Starting at the outer corners, sweep a darker, matte shade into the crease and along the lower lash line. If desired, use a sparkly, light nude shade to highlight the inner corners of the eyes. Line the top lash line with black gel or pencil eyeliner and extend the line past the outer corners to make the eyes appear larger. Finish the look with black mascara on both the top and bottom lashes.

TIP: *Foundation brushes are great for getting into small corners of the face, and they allow you to "tap" layers where needed.*

CHEEKS & LIPS: Apply a rosy champagne cheek color along the hollows of the cheeks, then blend upwards to give dimension to the face. Dust whatever is left on your cheek brush onto your temples. Perfect your lip shape with a lip liner, then swipe a golden, chocolate-brown lipstick all over your lips. Repeat for extra staying power!

SELFIE TIP:
Dry, flaky skin always shows up on selfies!
Make sure your lips are smooth and soft before you apply a
bold lip color by exfoliating and moisturizing them first.

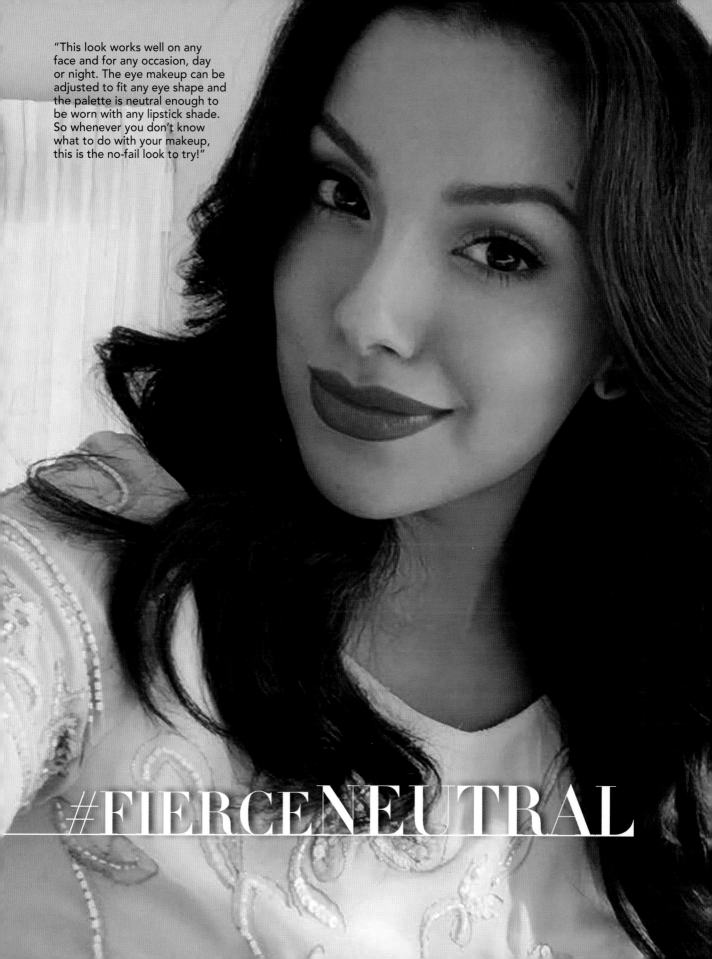

"This look works well on any face and for any occasion, day or night. The eye makeup can be adjusted to fit any eye shape and the palette is neutral enough to be worn with any lipstick shade. So whenever you don't know what to do with your makeup, this is the no-fail look to try!"

#FIERCENEUTRAL

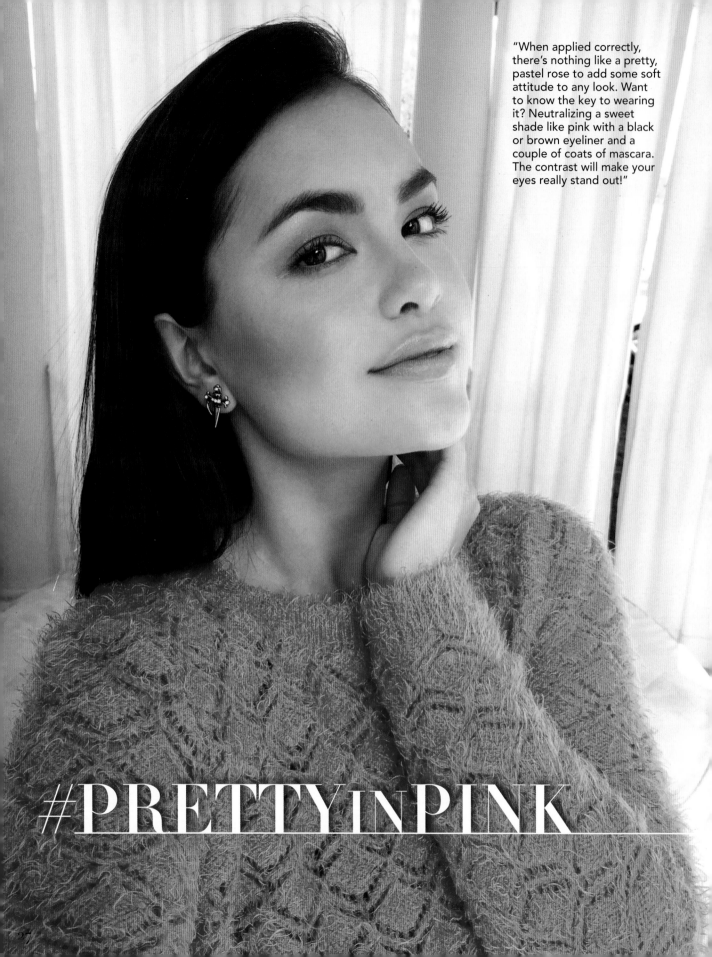

"When applied correctly, there's nothing like a pretty, pastel rose to add some soft attitude to any look. Want to know the key to wearing it? Neutralizing a sweet shade like pink with a black or brown eyeliner and a couple of coats of mascara. The contrast will make your eyes really stand out!"

#PRETTYinPINK

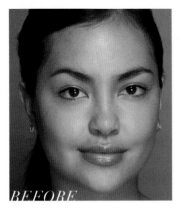

BEFORE

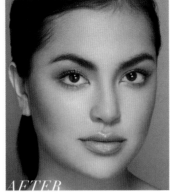

AFTER

The Essentials

- Soft pink and light nude matte eyeshadows
- Eyeshadow, smudger and cheek brushes
- Mascara
- Bronzer
- Warm peach cheek color
- Pink lipstick

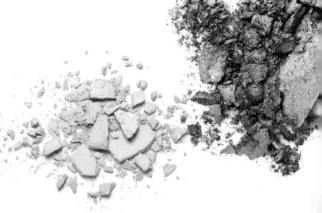

one

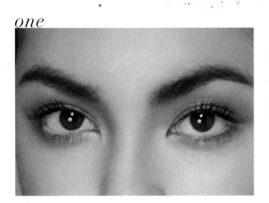

EYES: Dust a soft pink eyeshadow over the eyelid and right above the crease. Take a smudger brush (the kind with short bristles in a tight shape) and lightly line the lower lash line with the pink eyeshadow, from corner to corner. Blend well. With a clean, fluffy eyeshadow brush, blend away any visible edges. For an eye-brightening appearance, highlight the brow bone with a light nude matte eyeshadow. Curl your lashes and apply a coat of mascara.

TIP: *If you have small or hooded eyelids, you can check your eyeshadow application by looking straight into a mirror — you should be able to see the shadow right above your crease.*

CHEEKS & LIPS: Dot a sheer pink lipstick onto your lips with your fingertips, working from the outer corners in. Sculpt the cheeks with bronzer and blend well. Lightly dust a slightly shimmery pink cheek color over the bronzer.

two

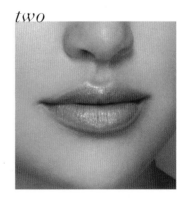

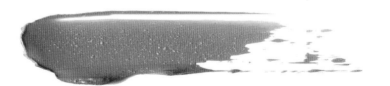

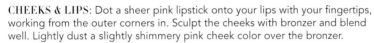

SELFIE TIP:
Try wearing a top with texture. It will add interest to your selfies without being distracting.

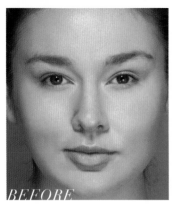
BEFORE

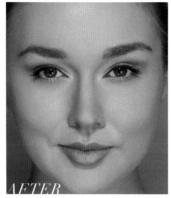
AFTER

The Essentials

- Foundation or tinted moisturizer
- Bone, pink-brown and black eyeshadows
- Mascara
- Eyeliner or smudger brush
- Rosy peach cheek color
- Creamy lipstick in a natural peach shade

one

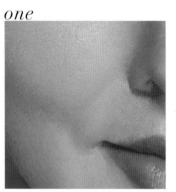

two

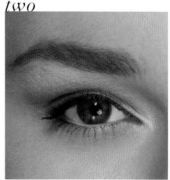

three

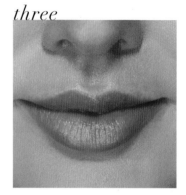

SKIN: Apply foundation or tinted moisturizer to already moisturized skin. Make sure it's blended well so there are no visible lines.

TIP: *To determine which shade of foundation best matches your skin tone, test it on your jawline instead of the back of your hand. Stand by a window to see how the shade looks in natural light.*

EYES: Starting at the inner corners of your eyes, apply a natural-looking, bone shade of eyeshadow all over your eyelids. Contour the crease with a pink-brown shade, then blend. With an eyeliner or smudger brush, apply a thin line of black eyeshadow along the upper lashes. Extend the line past the outer corner and flick it out slightly into a cat-eye, if desired. Finish with two coats of mascara.

CHEEKS & LIPS: Apply a rosy peach blush to the apples of the cheeks, then apply bronzer to the hollows of the cheeks, along the hairline and under the jawline. Blend the blush and bronzer together well. After exfoliating and moisturizing your lips, swipe on a creamy lipstick in a natural peach shade.

TIP: *For a natural look, swipe the lipstick onto the bottom lip and press the lips together. Repeat for a long-lasting effect.*

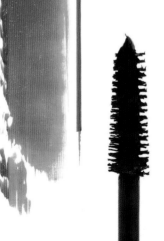

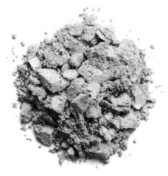

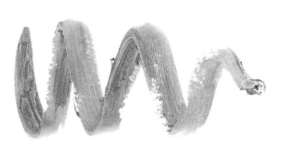

SELFIE TIP:
A fake smile is never flattering. Be genuine while taking your selfies! Think of something funny or that makes you truly happy and snap away. You will see the difference.

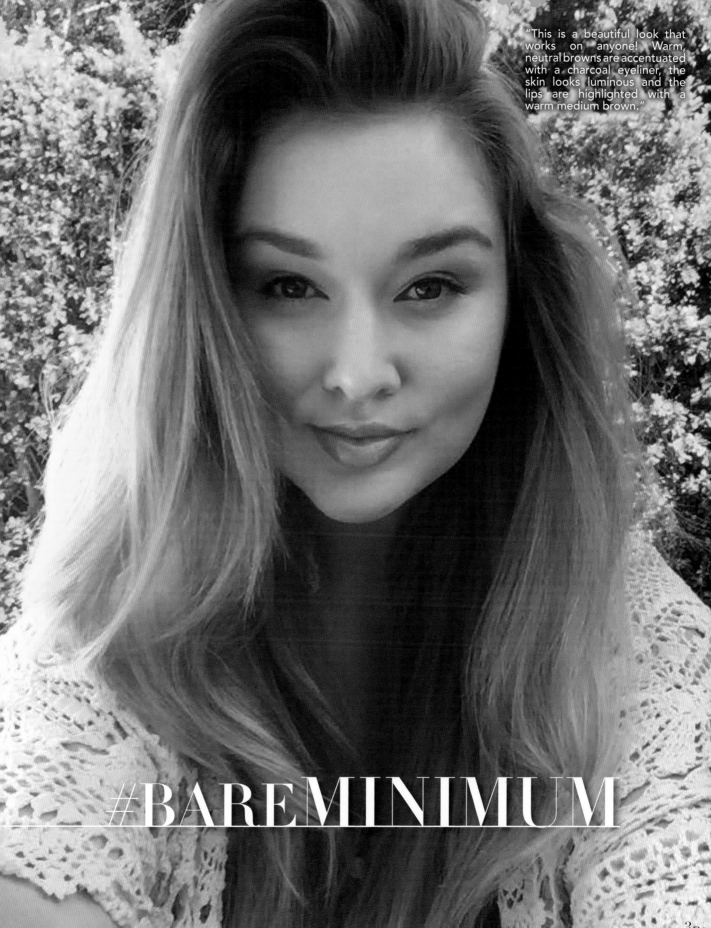

"This is a beautiful look that works on anyone! Warm, neutral browns are accentuated with a charcoal eyeliner, the skin looks luminous and the lips are highlighted with a warm medium brown."

#BAREMINIMUM

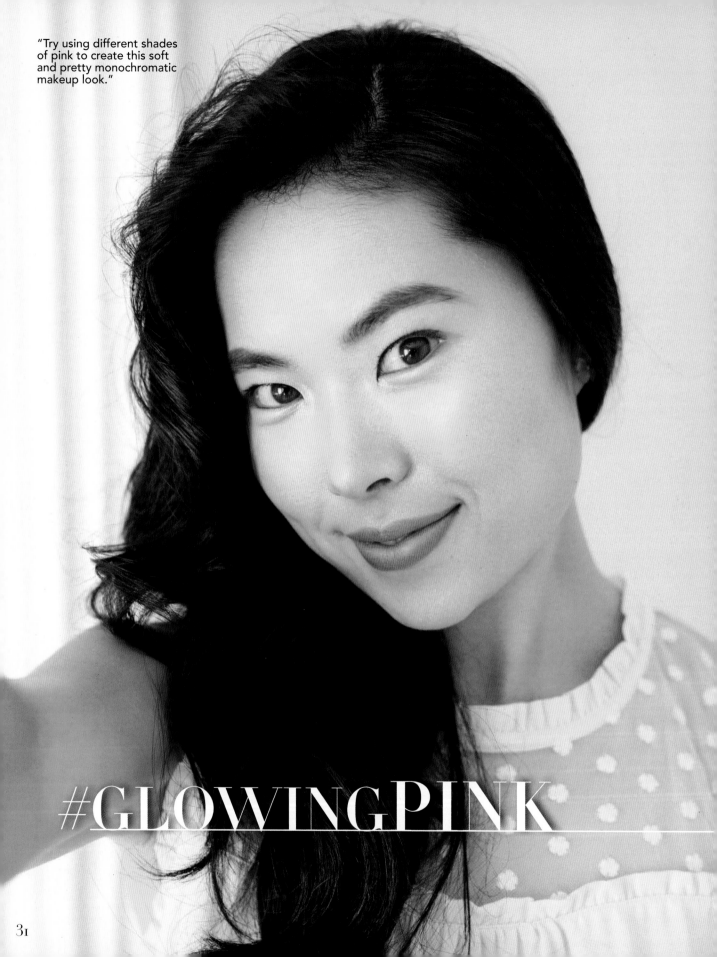

"Try using different shades of pink to create this soft and pretty monochromatic makeup look."

#GLOWINGPINK

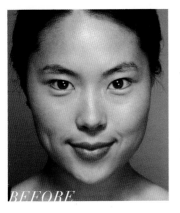

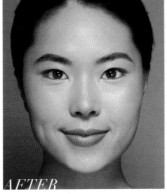

BEFORE *AFTER*

The Essentials

- Eyeshadows in golden pink, soft pink and creamy pearl shades
- Soft coral or rose cheek color
- Sheer coral cheek color
- Slightly iridescent powder highlighter
- Lip exfoliator and lip balm
- Creamy pink lipstick

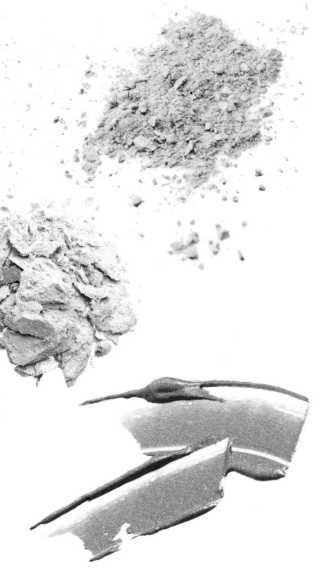

one

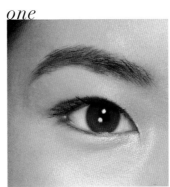

two

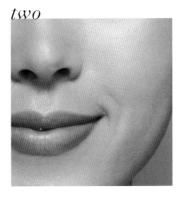

EYES: For this look, you'll be creating what is called a "gradient color technique" — a pink ombré eyeshadow effect from your lash line to your brows. Start by applying the golden pink eyeshadow to your lash line and eyelids with an eyeshadow brush. Next, dust the soft pink shadow onto the crease. Finish by applying the creamy pearl shade onto the brow bone and the inner corners of the eyes.

TIP: *The gradient technique works very well on hooded eyes.*

CHEEKS & LIPS: Using a high concentration of sheer coral blush on your blush brush, dust the blush onto your face, starting near your ears and softly swiping forward, under and slightly above the cheeks. To create a healthy sheen, apply a powder highlighter onto the upper portion of cheeks, the bridge of the nose and any other areas you want to accentuate.

Exfoliate your lips and apply balm to prep. Let the balm do its job while you put on the rest of your makeup, then apply a sheer pink lipstick either straight from the tube or with your fingertips.

SELFIE TIP:
Want full, sexy hair in seconds for your selfie? It's easy — just sweep it over one shoulder and voilà!

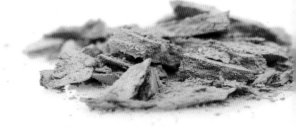

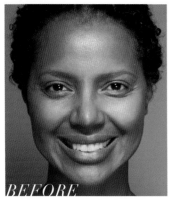

BEFORE

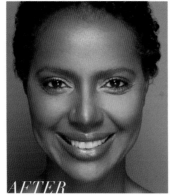

AFTER

The Essentials

- Two foundations: one a shade darker and one that matches your skin tone
- Two foundation brushes
- Kabuki brush or blending sponge
- Large powder brush
- Gold eyeshadow
- Almond-brown eyeshadow
- Black eyeliner
- Golden bronze lip gloss

one

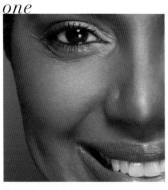

SKIN: Moisturize the skin and apply eye cream. Follow with a foundation primer. Using a foundation brush and starting at the top of your hairline, apply a foundation that is one shade darker than your skin tone. Move down along your hairline and curve around the hollows of the cheeks. Do the same along the sides of the nose and under the jawline. Next, take a foundation that matches your skin tone and apply it to the middle of the forehead, the bridge of the nose and in an inverted-V underneath the eyes. Blend the foundations together with a clean kabuki brush or a wet blending sponge. Follow with a golden coral cheek color, and finish by applying a colorless translucent powder all over the face with a large powder brush.

TIP: *The delicate under-eye area is usually the first spot on your face to show signs of aging, so make sure to take care of it and use eye cream daily.*

two

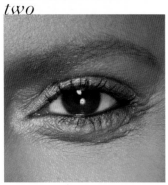

EYES: With a damp eyeshadow brush, apply gold eyeshadow to the inner corners of the eyes, then swipe the gold eyeshadow from your lid to just below your crease. Enhance the crease and outer corners by applying an almond-brown eyeshadow on top with a dry brush. Line the waterline with a clean, black eyeliner and finish with two coats of mascara on both top and bottom lashes.

TIP: *"Tightlining" the waterline makes eyes really pop. Make sure to always sanitize the tip of the eyeliner before using it to tightline and do not use that eyeliner on any other parts of the eye.*

three

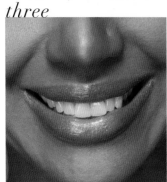

LIPS: Brush a tiny bit of foundation onto your lips to neutralize any discoloration. Then, apply a golden bronze lip gloss for a pretty and natural shine.

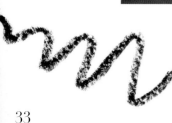

SELFIE TIP:
Loving your makeup today? Look straight into the camera and smile when you take your selfie. Confidence is one of your most beautiful assets!

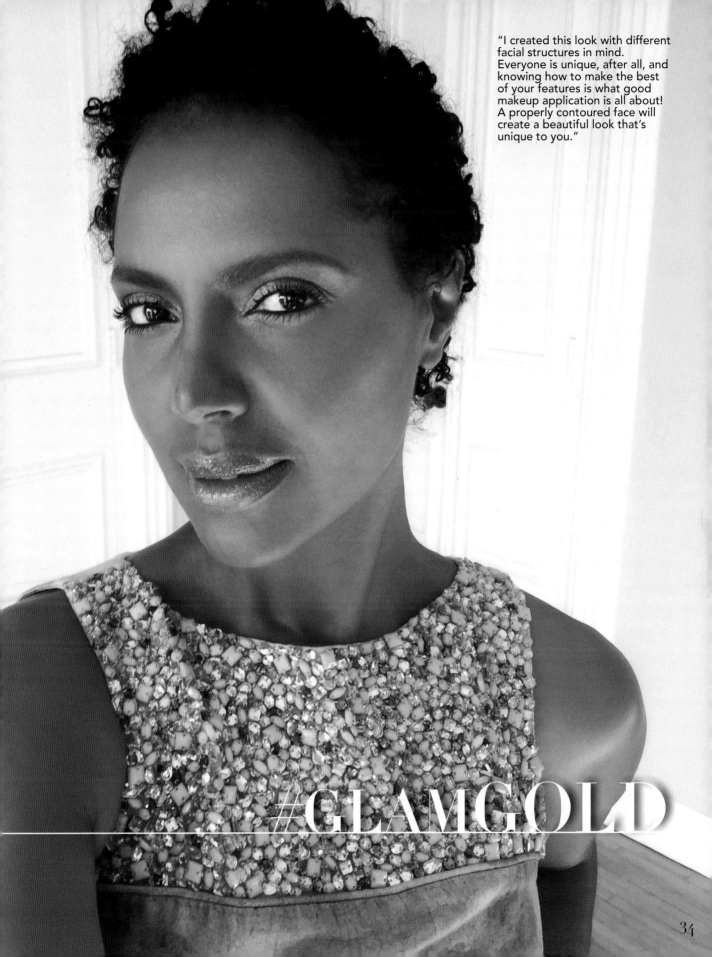

"I created this look with different facial structures in mind. Everyone is unique, after all, and knowing how to make the best of your features is what good makeup application is all about! A properly contoured face will create a beautiful look that's unique to you."

#GLAMGOLD

34

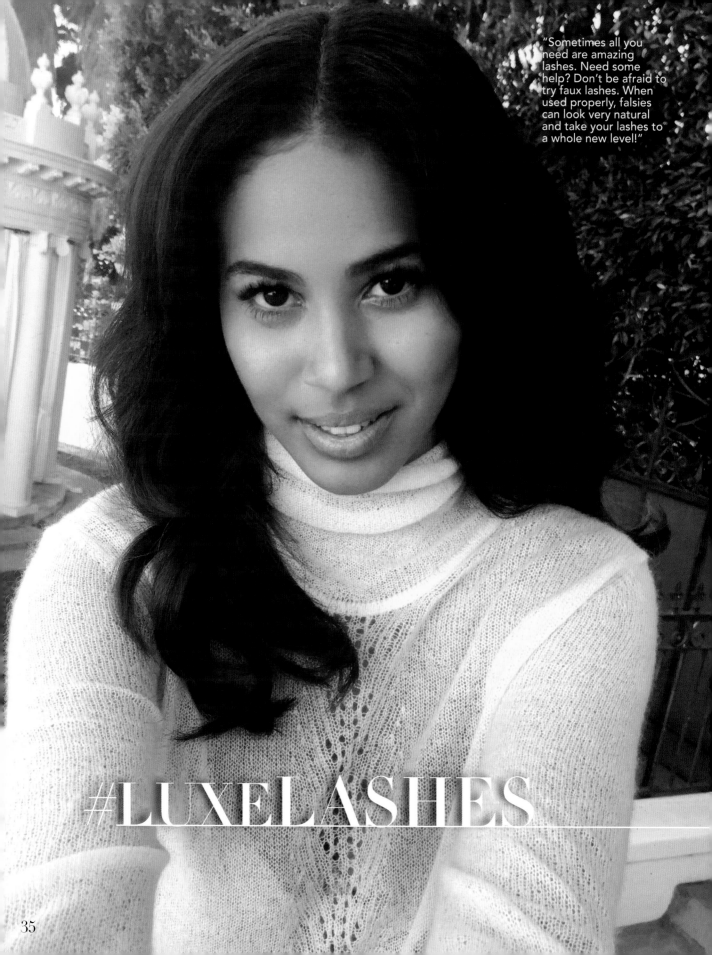

"Sometimes all you need are amazing lashes. Need some help? Don't be afraid to try faux lashes. When used properly, falsies can look very natural and take your lashes to a whole new level!"

#LUXELASHES

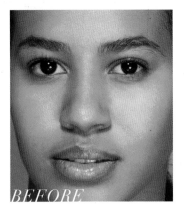

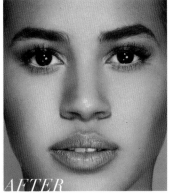

BEFORE   *AFTER*

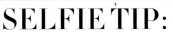

The Essentials

- Nude eyeshadow
- Dark brown and light brown eyeshadows
- Taupe eyeshadow in a shade slightly lighter than your skin tone
- Gel eyeliner
- Individual false lashes
- Lash glue
- Tweezers
- Mascara
- Golden bronze cheek color
- Sheer nude lipstick

one

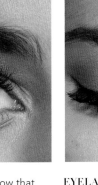

two

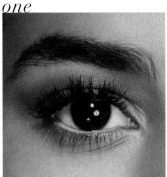

three

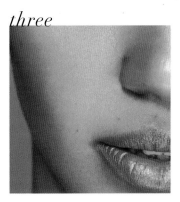

EYES: Dust an eyeshadow that is slightly lighter than your skin tone onto the entire lid from lash to brow bone. Starting at the outer corners of the eyes, sweep a dark brown matte shade onto the crease. Use a lighter brown eyeshadow on the crease to blend the darker shade, then carry it under the lower lash line.

EYELASHES: Curl your natural lashes and apply one coat of mascara. Apply the individual false lashes, alternating between short and medium lengths. Place lash glue on a clean surface and dip each eyelash lightly into the glue with a pair of tweezers. Let dry for about 30 seconds, until the glue becomes tacky. Starting at the inner corner of the eye, place a short cluster of lashes as close to the lash line as possible. Adjust the placement if necessary. Continue placing the lashes, one next to the other, all the way across the lash line. Wait until the glue has fully dried before applying another coat of mascara. If desired, apply a thin line of gel eyeliner to cover any visible application lines.

TIP: *For an elongated cat-eye effect, add extra lashes to the outer corners of each eye. For a fluttery round look, apply the longest clusters of lashes to the middle of the eyes, right above the iris.*

CHEEKS & LIPS: Dust a bronzer or warm gold blush onto the cheeks and pair it with a nude or neutral lipstick.

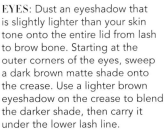

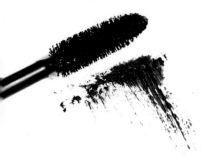

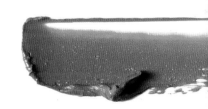

SELFIE TIP:
Individual faux lashes look more natural than full strips because you can better control placement and use different lengths. I use them often on my clients.

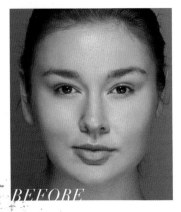

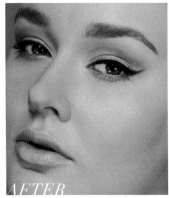

BEFORE *AFTER*

The Essentials

- Foundation
- Foundation brush
- Translucent powder
- Warm golden cheek color
- Bronzer
- Golden-pink, copper-gold, and brown eyeshadows
- Black gel eyeliner
- Angled eyeliner brush
- Sheer nude lipstick
- Natural shade of lip gloss
- Blotting papers

one

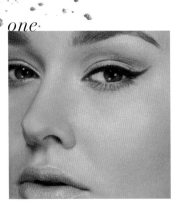

two

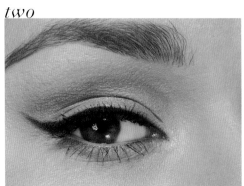

three

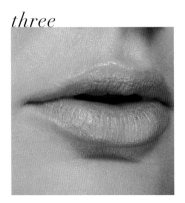

SKIN: Moisturize your face and wait a few minutes before applying a primer. Primer is not a must but it will make your makeup look better and stay put longer! Dot foundation onto the cheeks, nose and forehead. Blend with a foundation brush, using downward strokes. If you have oily skin, use a matte foundation and only apply powder where you need it most.

EYES: Brush a golden pink eyeshadow onto the lids, then apply a matte brown eyeshadow from the crease to the lower lash line. Use a copper-gold shadow to blend the brown shade away from the crease.

EYELINER: Use a gel eyeliner and angled brush to create your winged line. Starting close to the lower lash line at the outer corner of the eye, draw a diagonal line that follows the natural upward curve of the bottom lash line. Stop halfway between the end of your eyebrow and your eye's inner corner, then draw a straight line back to middle of the eyelid (you decide how thick you want it to be). Then, starting at the inner corner of the eye, draw a line to the outer corner, staying as close as possible to the lashes and thickening the line slightly as you go out. Continue by filling in the winged shape that's been created, making sure there aren't any gaps. Follow with mascara.

TIP: *If you need more help shaping your wing, try tracing the eyeliner along an imaginary, upturned line that follows the side of your eye and lower lash line.*

CHEEKS & LIPS: Using a cheek brush, sweep a warm golden blush onto the apples of the cheeks, blending up and out towards the ears. Add highlighter along the top of the cheekbones to accentuate, and if desired, a darker blush or bronzer along the cheek hollows to sculpt. Finish with a sheer nude lipstick and lip gloss.

TIP: *If you want to make your lip color matte, use oil-blotting papers! They will absorb the shine without removing pigment from your lips.*

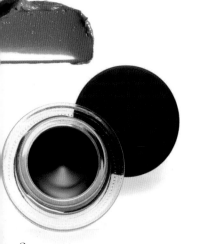

SELFIE TIP:
Finding the right shade of foundation is important. Always test a new shade by taking a selfie in natural light to make sure the makeup completely disappears into your skin.

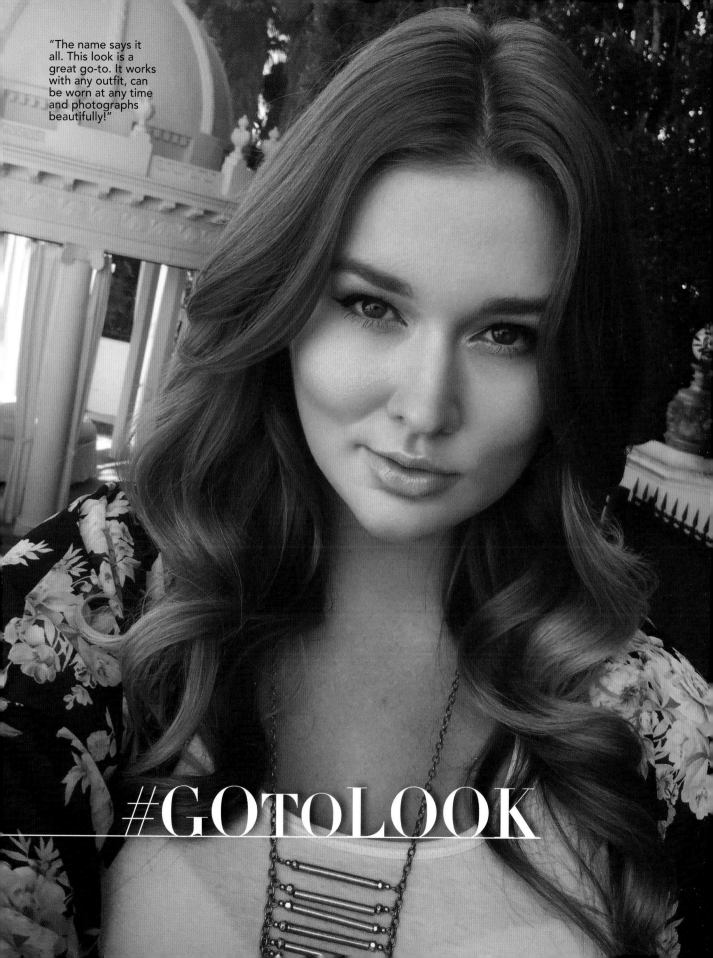

"The name says it all. This look is a great go-to. It works with any outfit, can be worn at any time and photographs beautifully!"

#GOTOLOOK

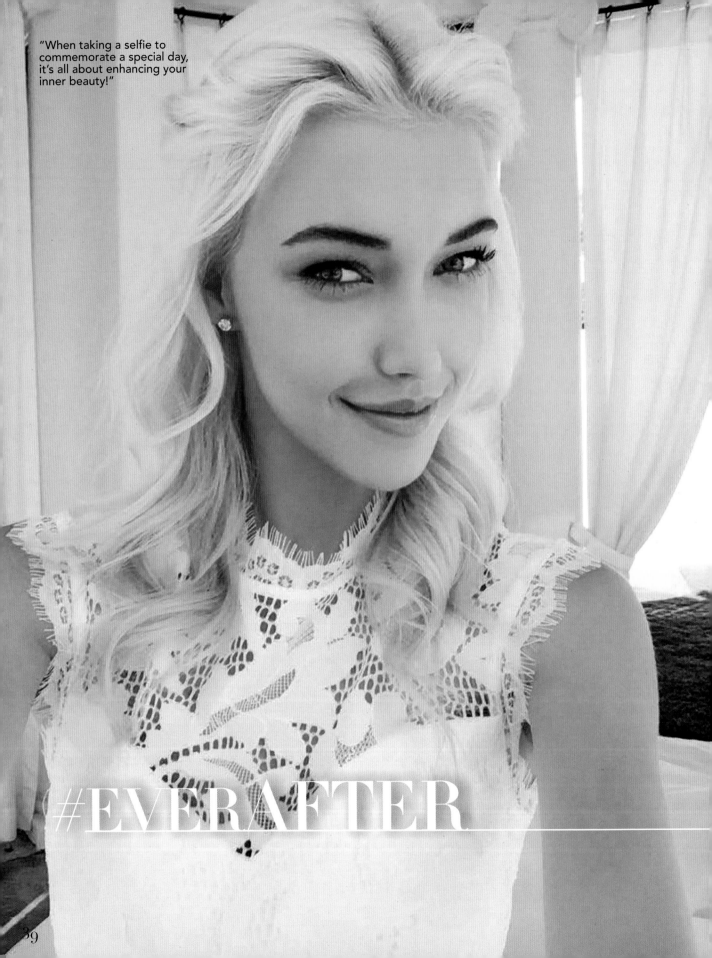

"When taking a selfie to commemorate a special day, it's all about enhancing your inner beauty!"

#EVERAFTER

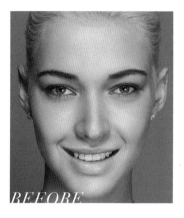

BEFORE

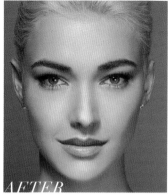

AFTER

The Essentials

- Matte foundation
- Translucent powder
- Concealer one shade lighter than your skin tone
- Blotting papers
- Eye smudger brush
- Eyeshadows in pearl, silver-gray and black
- Mascara
- Lip liner
- Golden pink cheek and lip colors
- Lip brush

one

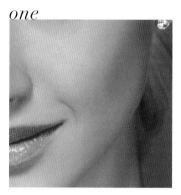

two

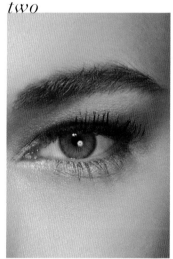

EYES: Smooth eye primer onto your lids and let dry. Apply light pearl eyeshadow from the inner corners of the eye up to the crease. Dust the same shade along the lower lash line. Apply a silver-gray eyeshadow to the crease to create depth, making sure to blend both shades thoroughly with a clean blending brush.

EYELINER & EYELASHES: Using a smudger brush, apply black eyeshadow to the base of the upper eyelashes by pressing it into a smooth line. Blend slightly for a smoky effect. Finish with two coats of waterproof mascara in black.

three

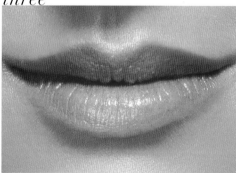

SKIN: Smooth primer onto clean, moisturized skin. Dot matte foundation onto the center of your face and blend outwards where needed, including the neck. Apply a concealer that's a little lighter than your skin tone to the under-eye area. Using a large powder brush, dust the face with translucent powder. Carry blotting papers in your purse to use for touch-ups during your event. They absorb oil without disturbing your makeup and keep your skin looking fresh.

TIP: _Use a concealer brush to cover flaws in small areas like the inner corners of the eyes and the sides of the nose.._

CHEEKS & LIPS: Apply a golden peach blush to the apples of the cheeks and blend. Line the lips with a liner pencil that matches your skin tone or is one shade darker. Using a lip brush, apply two coats of sheer pink lipstick, blotting in between coats for a long-lasting effect.

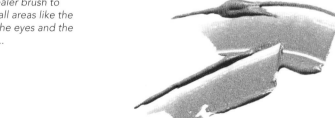

SELFIE TIP:

The subtleties! When posing for your selfies, it's all about the small details. After each shot, try moving slowly and making tiny changes. Moving your chin up or down or slightly parting your lips are small movements that can really create the best results!

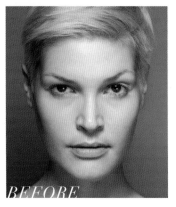

BEFORE

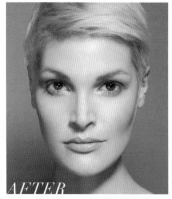

AFTER

The Essentials

- Eyeshadow in light gold, peach-pink and soft blue shades
- Three clean eyeshadow brushes
- Slightly sparkly peach-pink cheek color
- Lengthening mascara
- Neutral lip liner
- Creamy lipstick one shade darker than your natural lip color

one

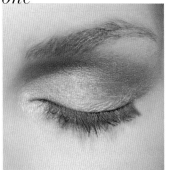

two

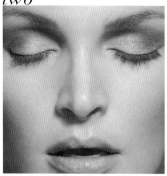

three

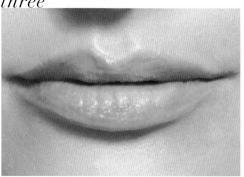

EYES: With an eyeshadow brush, dust a light gold eyeshadow onto the eyelid from the inner corner to the middle of the lid. Using another brush, apply the peach-pink eyeshadow to the outer third of the eye and shade along the crease. Use another clean brush to blend. Starting at the outer corners, dust a light blue eyeshadow over to the crease and along lower lash line. Blend thoroughly to soften the color. Curl the lashes and apply mascara to the top lashes only.

TIP: *Blending a light shade of eyeshadow into the inner corners of the eyes brightens and helps to bring out smaller eyes.*

CHEEKS: For a quick and youthful-looking lift, dust a slightly sparkly, salmon-peach blush onto the highest points of the cheeks.

TIP: *How do you know which shade of blush is best for you? Think of the color your cheeks turn when you're naturally flushed or when you pinch them. Use the same shade of blush for the most natural hue.*

LIPS: Exfoliate and moisturize your lips, then follow with a neutral lip liner if desired. Finish the look with a creamy lipstick that's about one shade darker than your natural lip color.

SELFIE TIP:

Don't be afraid to take many shots of one look. There's nothing wrong with having a lot of options!

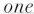

#COASTALBLUES

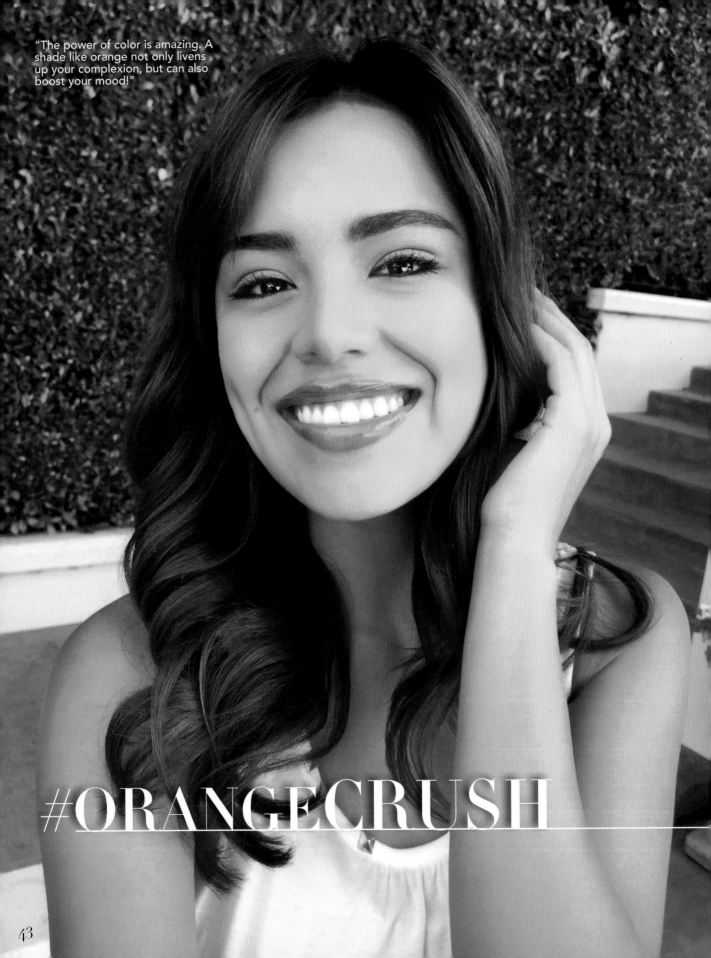

"The power of color is amazing. A shade like orange not only livens up your complexion, but can also boost your mood!"

#ORANGECRUSH

43

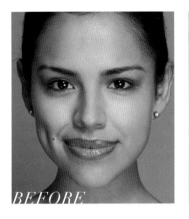
BEFORE

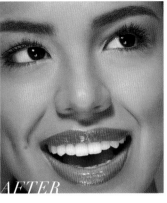
AFTER

The Essentials

- Gold-copper and light beige eyeshadow
- Bronzer
- Golden citrus cheek color
- Cheek brush
- Sheer apricot lipstick
- Warm orange lip gloss

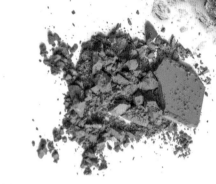

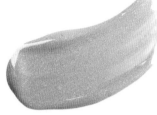

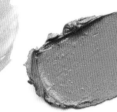

one

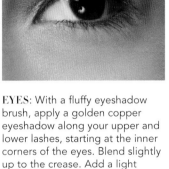

two

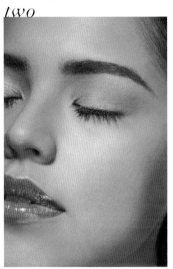

three

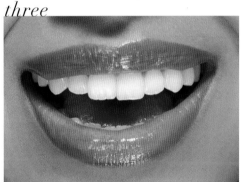

EYES: With a fluffy eyeshadow brush, apply a golden copper eyeshadow along your upper and lower lashes, starting at the inner corners of the eyes. Blend slightly up to the crease. Add a light beige hue and blend from the crease to the brow bone. Finish off with two coats of mascara.

CHEEKS: With a cheek brush, apply bronzer to the temples, the hollows of the cheeks, underneath the jawline and any other area where the sun would naturally hit. Next, dust a golden citrus blush on top of your cheeks. Blend towards the hairline and into the bronzer.

TIP: *If you have very round cheeks, apply blush to the tops of the cheeks, about two finger widths from the side of the nose.*

LIPS: Beginning at the outer corners of the lips and working inwards, apply an apricot lipstick with your fingertips.

TIP: *This technique creates a pretty, stained look and is a great way to try wearing a color that might normally be too bright for you. Kick up the intensity by adding a warm orange lip gloss on top.*

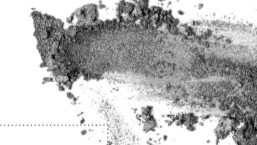

SELFIE TIP:

Clean your camera lens! Have you ever noticed a hazy look to your selfies? It's usually because the lens on your phone needs to be cleaned. Get some lens cleaning solution and a soft cloth — it will make a difference!

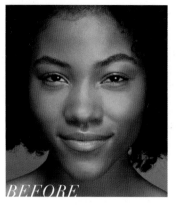
BEFORE

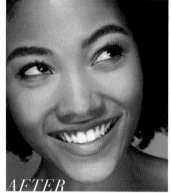
AFTER

The Essentials

- Tinted moisturizer, CC or BB cream
- Translucent powder
- Blotting papers
- Warm gold eyeshadow stick or chubby pencil
- Copper-brown and purple eyeliners
- Berry colored lip and cheek stick

one

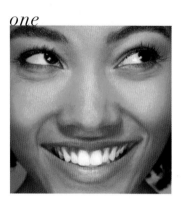

two

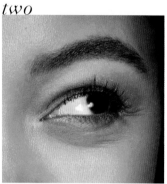

three

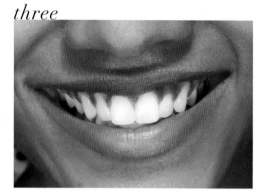

SKIN: Use a tinted moisturizer, BB or CC cream with SPF to correct any imperfections and even out skin tone. Set with powder, if needed, but if you have oily skin, use sparingly. Carry blotting papers with you instead to dab off excess moisture and oil throughout the day.

EYES: Using a shadow stick or chubby pencil, create a warm gold base over the eyelid. Line the eyes along the top lashes with a coppery brown chubby eyeliner pencil, then slightly smudge the line with your fingers at the outer corners. Draw a very thin line of purple along the lower lash line for a pop of color. Finish the eyes with a couple of coats of mascara.

TIP: *Adding a brightly colored eyeliner to the bottom lash line is an easy way to make a statement!*

CHEEKS & LIPS: Apply a creamy cheek color to the apples of the cheeks and dab the same shade onto the lips.

TIP: *Two-in-one cheek and lip duos are great, but in a pinch, lipstick alone can work on both the cheeks and lips.*

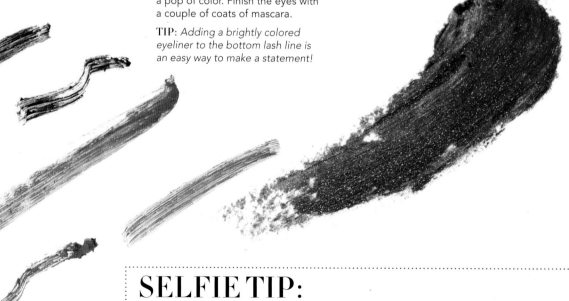

SELFIE TIP:

An easy way to express different emotions in your selfies is to change up the direction of your eyes. A side view with a smile, for example, looks fun and youthful!

#COLORPLAY

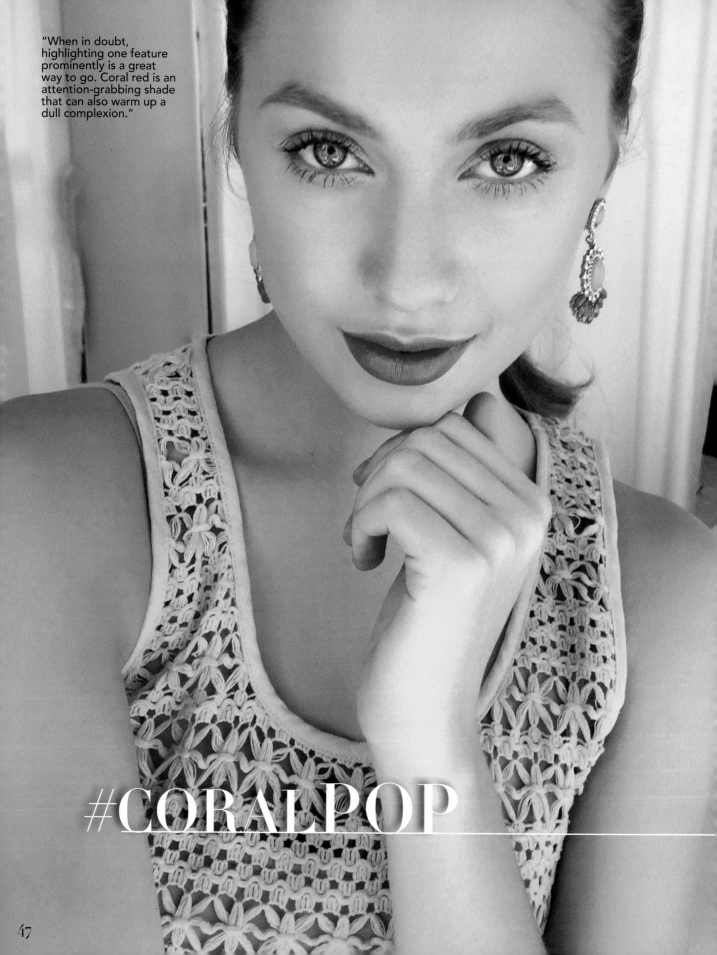

"When in doubt, highlighting one feature prominently is a great way to go. Coral red is an attention-grabbing shade that can also warm up a dull complexion."

#CORALPOP

47

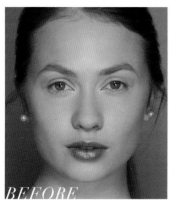

BEFORE

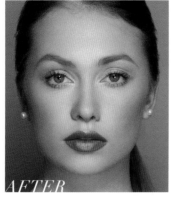

AFTER

The Essentials

- Foundation
- Concealer
- Translucent powder
- Eyebrow pencil
- Eyebrow gel
- Warm orange lip gloss
- Matte brown eyeshadow
- Shimmery gold cream eyeshadow
- Warm gold eyeshadow
- Mascara
- Cheek and lip tint in orange-red
- Neutral lip liner

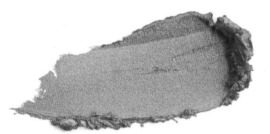

one

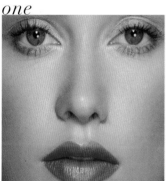

two

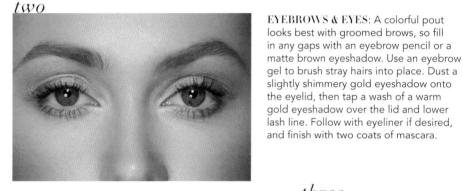

EYEBROWS & EYES: A colorful pout looks best with groomed brows, so fill in any gaps with an eyebrow pencil or a matte brown eyeshadow. Use an eyebrow gel to brush stray hairs into place. Dust a slightly shimmery gold eyeshadow onto the eyelid, then tap a wash of a warm gold eyeshadow over the lid and lower lash line. Follow with eyeliner if desired, and finish with two coats of mascara.

SKIN: Apply primer to clean, moisturized skin. Follow with foundation, concealer and a dusting of translucent powder.

TIP: *Choose a primer with light-diffusing particles to help even and perfect your skin tone.*

LIPS: Don't be afraid of brightly colored lip colors! Look for a combination lip-and-cheek product or a powder blush in the same shade as your orange-red lipstick. Place a couple of dots of orange-red lip color onto the apples of your cheeks, then use a sponge to blend. Apply the same shade to your lips with your ring finger. Blot and reapply. Line lips with a neutral shade if necessary.

TIP: *If you think the bright shade may look too bold, mix it with a bit of foundation on the back of your hand before you apply. This will subdue the strong color and create a sheer, natural effect.*

three

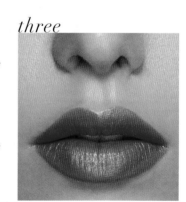

SELFIE TIP:

Check that focus! Touch the part of the picture you want to focus on (I like to use the eyes on a selfie) to ensure that the image is nice and clear.

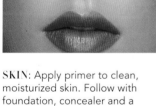

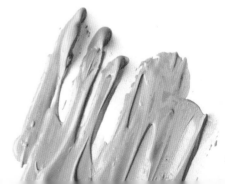

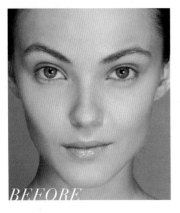

BEFORE

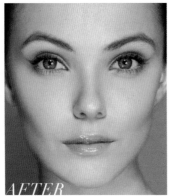

AFTER

The Essentials

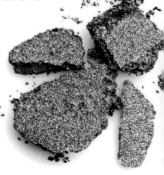

- Light plum and violet eyeshadows
- Angled eyeliner brush
- Berry-bronze cheek color
- Gold-pink lip gloss

one

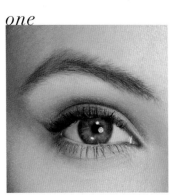

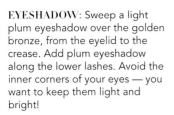

two

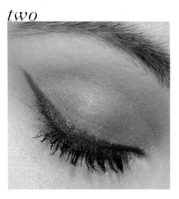

three

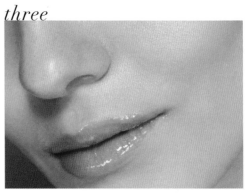

EYESHADOW: Sweep a light plum eyeshadow over the golden bronze, from the eyelid to the crease. Add plum eyeshadow along the lower lashes. Avoid the inner corners of your eyes — you want to keep them light and bright!

EYELINER: Dip a damp angled eyeliner brush into a corner of the violet eyeshadow pan. Before you apply, test the shade's consistency and intensity on the back of your hand. You want a creamy texture that glides easily and a color that is bright. Place your finger just above your cheekbone and pull lightly in a downward direction to keep your skin taut while you apply. Start at the inner corner and move across the lash line, thickening the line as you move towards the middle. When you reach the outer corner of the eye, create a slight flick. Go over the line once more, if necessary. Finish by curling the lashes and adding two coats of mascara.

TIP: *Avoid smears and smudges by allowing the eyeliner to dry thoroughly before opening your eyes too wide.*

CHEEKS & LIPS: Apply a warm berry-bronze cheek color over pink blush to accentuate the cheeks. Finish by dabbing on a gold-pink lip gloss.

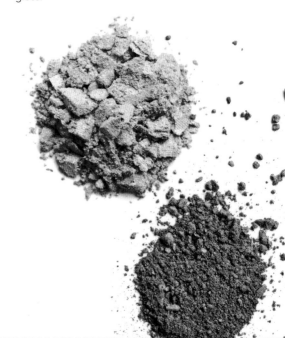

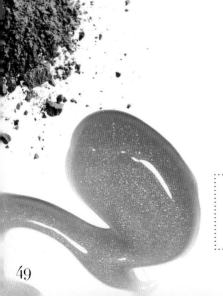

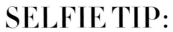

SELFIE TIP:

Want to make your eyes look bigger in your selfies? Angle the camera up high and shoot from above.

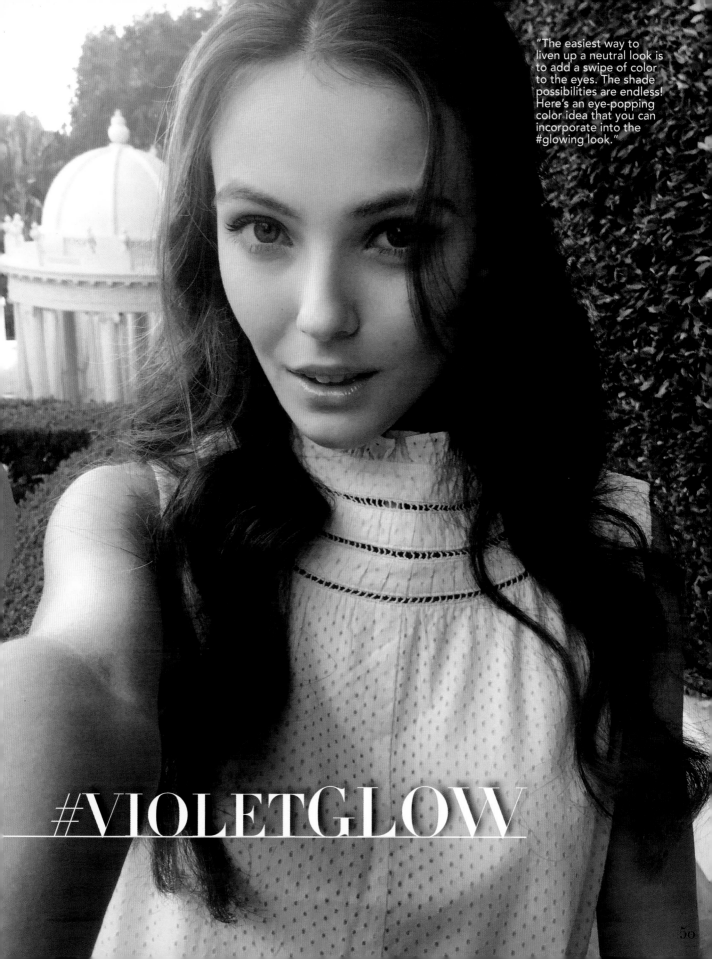

"The easiest way to liven up a neutral look is to add a swipe of color to the eyes. The shade possibilities are endless! Here's an eye-popping color idea that you can incorporate into the #glowing look."

#VIOLETGLOW

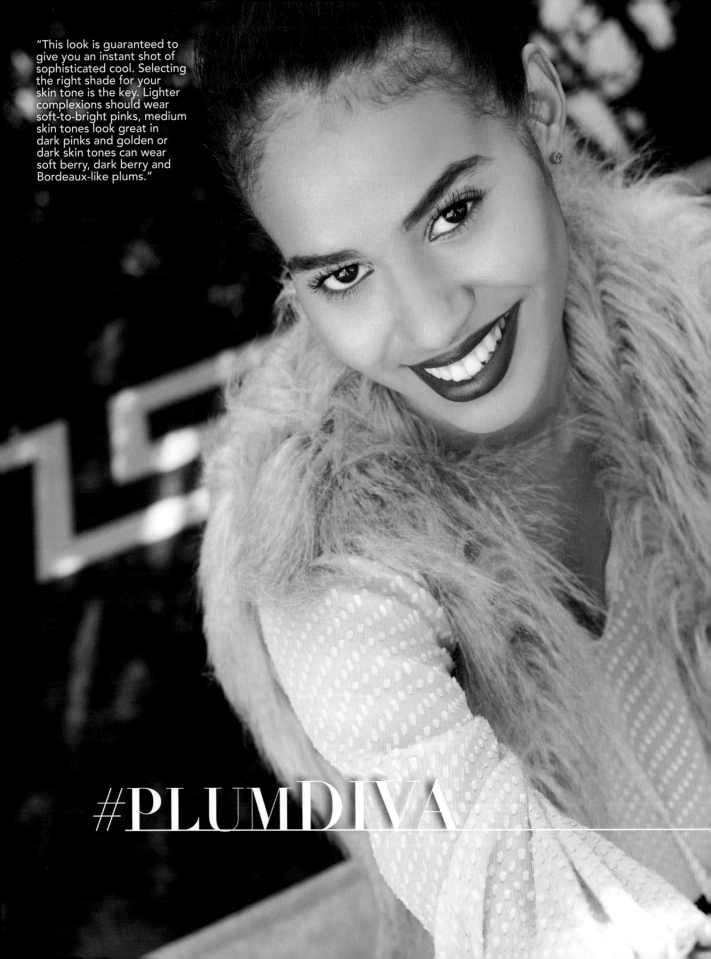

"This look is guaranteed to give you an instant shot of sophisticated cool. Selecting the right shade for your skin tone is the key. Lighter complexions should wear soft-to-bright pinks, medium skin tones look great in dark pinks and golden or dark skin tones can wear soft berry, dark berry and Bordeaux-like plums."

#PLUMDIVA

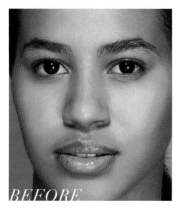
BEFORE

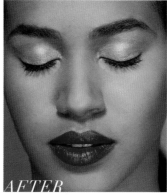
AFTER

The Essentials

- Eyebrow pencil
- Eyebrow gel
- Pearl colored cream eyeshadow or iridescent pearl powder eyeshadow
- Steel-gray powder eyeshadow
- Lip exfoliator
- Lip balm
- Lip liner
- Plum lipstick
- Mascara

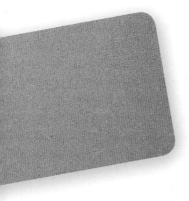

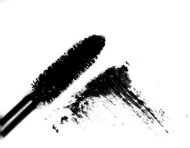

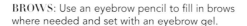

one

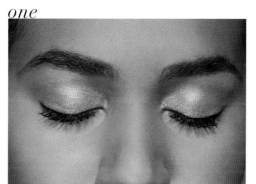

two

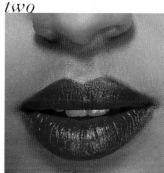

BROWS: Use an eyebrow pencil to fill in brows where needed and set with an eyebrow gel.

TIP: *Don't make eyebrows too thin. Fuller brows are sexy and totally in!*

EYES: Give the eyes a simple glow by applying a pearl-colored cream eyeshadow to the lid. Next, apply a steel-gray powder eyeshadow from the lash line to the crease. Curl your lashes and apply two coats of mascara.

LIPS: It's crucial to exfoliate your lips prior to applying a dark lipstick. After sloughing off dead skin, apply balm and allow it to penetrate and moisturize the lips. After a few minutes, blot off any excess balm and apply a plum lipstick right from the tube.

TIP: *After applying lipstick, trace your lips with a lip liner to keep the color from bleeding and feathering.*

SELFIE TIP:

Don't be afraid to rock a bold, dark lip in your selfies! Remember that the glossier the lipstick, the easier it will be to wear (and photograph!). Go for a sheer lipstick or even a dark gloss if you are intimidated by a dark matte hue.

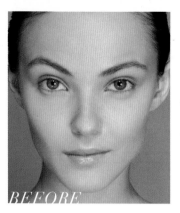

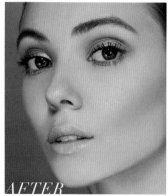

BEFORE

AFTER

The Essentials

- Light soft pink eyeshadow
- Silver eyeshadow
- Silver cream or pencil eyeshadow
- Eyeshadow brush
- Mascara
- Pearly pink cheek color
- Nude lip liner
- Nude lipstick
- Sparkly nude lip gloss

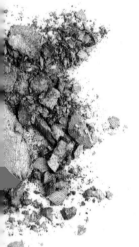

one

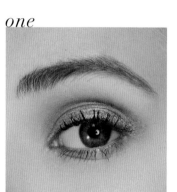

two

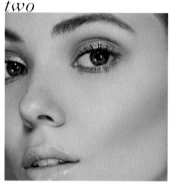

three

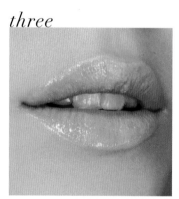

EYES: Dab an eye primer or concealer onto the eyelid. Using a fluffy eyeshadow brush, dust a soft pink eyeshadow from the lash line to just above the crease. Blend well. Draw a thin line of silver eyeshadow along the upper lash line with a stiff angled eyeliner brush, carrying the line to the outer corner. Curl your lashes, then brush on a couple of coats of mascara.

TIP: *Give your eyeliner maximum impact by starting with a layer of silver cream or pencil eyeshadow before applying the silver shade.*

CHEEKS: Give your cheeks a light glow by dusting on a pearly pink blush. Blend well into the hairline. Follow with a highlighter on the top of cheeks, the bridge of the nose and blended into the décolletage.

LIPS: Exfoliate and moisturize lips. Use a nude lip liner as a base to hold the color longer, then apply a light nude shade of lipstick on top. Finish with a sparkly nude gloss.

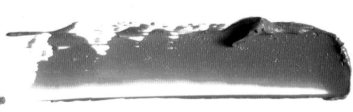

SELFIE TIP:
Remember to bring on the attitude! Use facial expressions and body language to let everyone know how you are feeling.

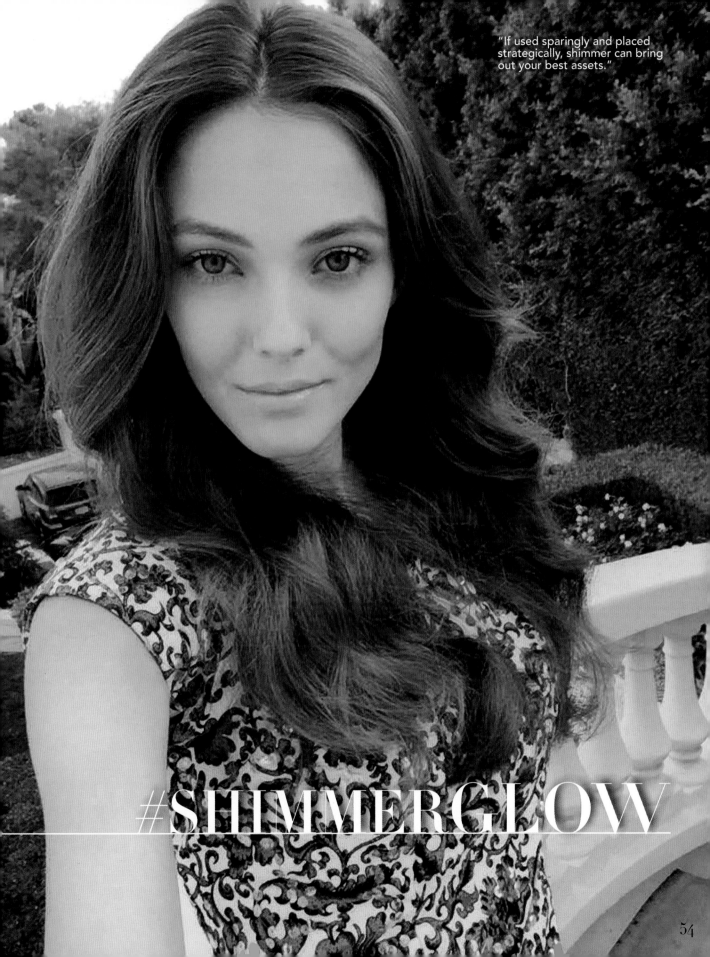

"If used sparingly and placed strategically, shimmer can bring out your best assets."

#SHIMMERGLOW

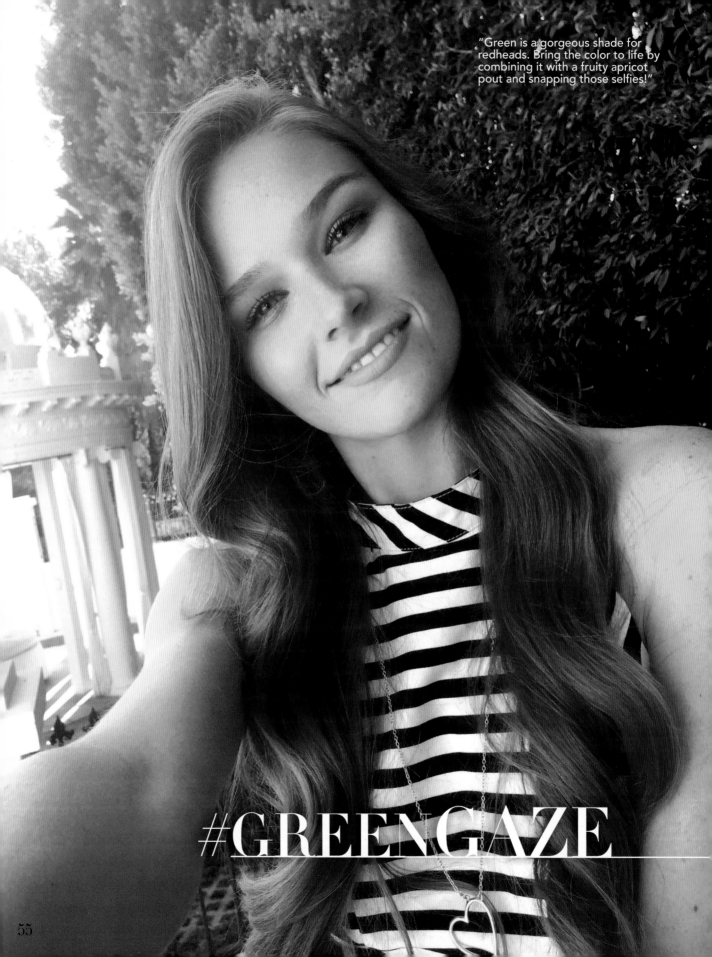

"Green is a gorgeous shade for redheads. Bring the color to life by combining it with a fruity apricot pout and snapping those selfies!"

#GREENGAZE

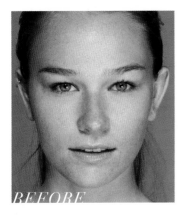

BEFORE

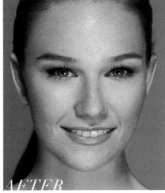

AFTER

The Essentials

- Tinted moisturizer or CC cream
- Concealer
- Light gold, lime-green and black eyeshadows
- Angled eyeliner brush
- Mascara
- Rosy cheek color
- Cheek brush
- Salmon-orange lipstick
- Neutral lip liner

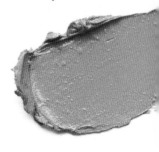

one

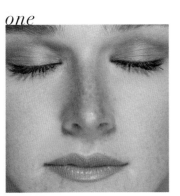

two

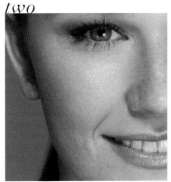

three

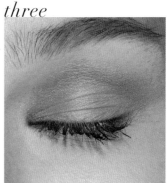

SKIN: With your fingertips, apply a thin layer of tinted moisturizer or CC cream to clean, moisturized skin. Work from the center of your face along the contours, the sides of the nose and the jawline until the cream is completely blended. Add a small amount of concealer where needed.

TIP: *There's no need to cake on a ton of foundation — if you have freckles, embrace them!*

CHEEKS: Apply a sparkling rosy blush onto the apples of the cheeks and blend upwards towards the ears with a cheek brush.

TIP: *Try forming a figure "8" over your cheeks when blending the blush.*

EYES: Starting at the inner corners of the eyes, dust a light gold eyeshadow onto the lid, up to the crease and along the lower lash line. Apply a lime-green shade and blend towards the brow bone with a clean blending brush. Staying as close to the lash line as possible, line the top lashes with black eyeshadow using an angled eyeliner brush. Curl your lashes and apply one or two coats of mascara.

four

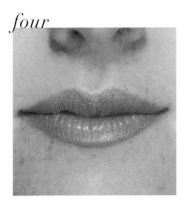

LIPS: Swipe a creamy, salmon lipstick onto the lips. Finish with a neutral lip liner, if necessary.

SELFIE TIP:
Don't forget your hair—it's an accessory! In this shot, the hair works perfectly with the makeup look.

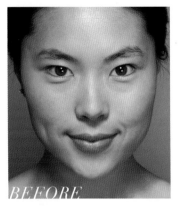
BEFORE

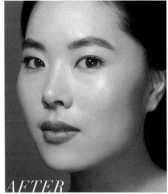
AFTER

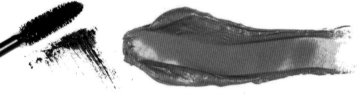

The Essentials

- Moisturizing mask
- Luminous foundation or mineral powder foundation
- Cream or powder highlighter
- Concealer
- Cream or silver-gray powder eyeshadow
- Light blue eyeshadow or eyeliner
- Stiff eyeliner brush
- Blush brush
- Eyelash curler
- Mascara
- Soft berry cheek and lip colors

one

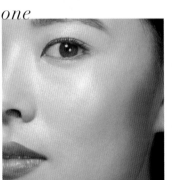

SKIN: Prep with a moisturizing mask to create a supple canvas for your makeup application. Add primer if desired, then apply a small amount of a luminous foundation or mineral powder foundation onto the face. The mineral foundation will give you nice, sheer coverage without feeling heavy. Concentrate on the areas where you need the most coverage. Follow by applying a cream or powder highlighter to the tops of the cheeks.

TIP: The slight sheen of the highlighter draws people's eyes up, making your cheekbones look higher.

three

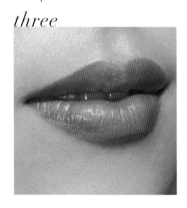

two

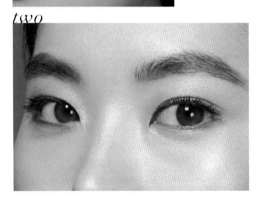

EYES: Apply concealer to your eyelids to serve as a brightening primer and under your eyes to correct any dark spots. Follow by dusting a silver-gray eyeshadow onto the lid, blending it to just above the crease. Do not apply eyeliner on the upper lash line. Using a stiff eyeliner brush, press a blue eyeshadow onto the bottom lash line, then blend downward as far as you feel comfortable. The smudged effect will add depth and make your eyes look larger. Curl your lashes well with an eyelash curler, squeezing them first at the base and again in the center to enhance the curve. A curler not only curls the lashes but also aligns the hairs so they appear thicker. Finish with two coats of black mascara.

TIP: Don't drag the blue color too far beneath your eyes — you don't want to create dark under-eye circles!

CHEEKS & LIPS: Apply a high concentration of blush near your ears and softly blend forward, under and slightly above the cheeks. For a healthy sheen, dust a powder highlighter onto the upper portion of cheeks, the bridge of the nose and to any other area you want to bring out. Finish with a swipe of sheer pink creamy lipstick.

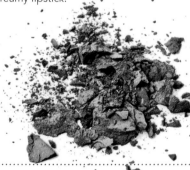

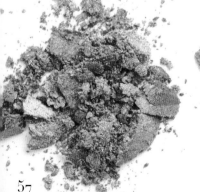

SELFIE TIP:
Relax and breathe. Holding your breath usually makes you look like... well, like you're holding your breath!

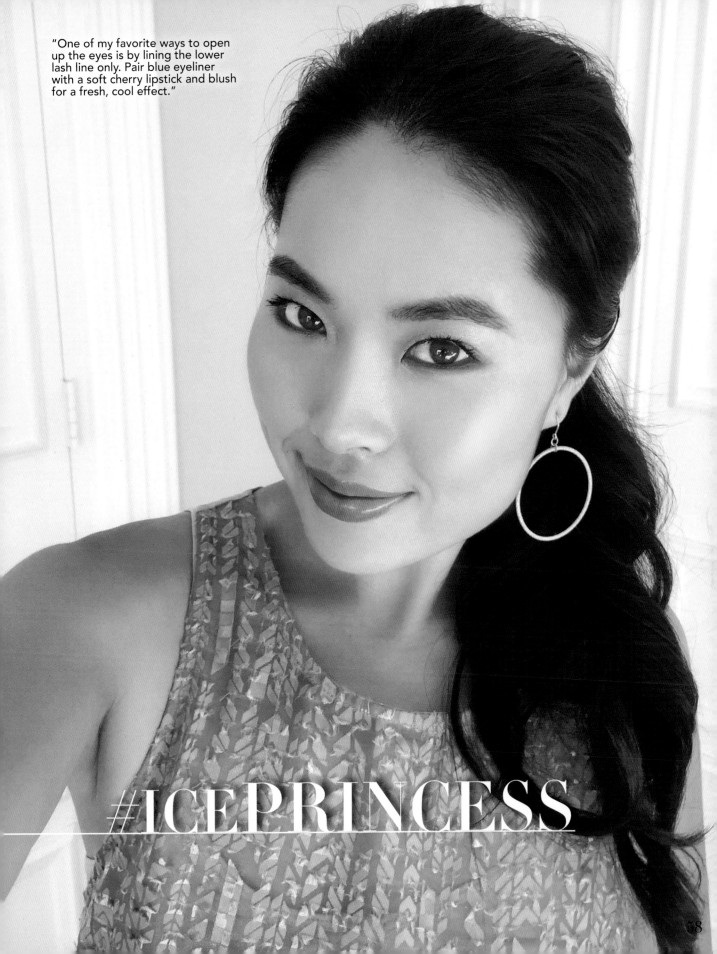

"One of my favorite ways to open up the eyes is by lining the lower lash line only. Pair blue eyeliner with a soft cherry lipstick and blush for a fresh, cool effect."

#ICEPRINCESS

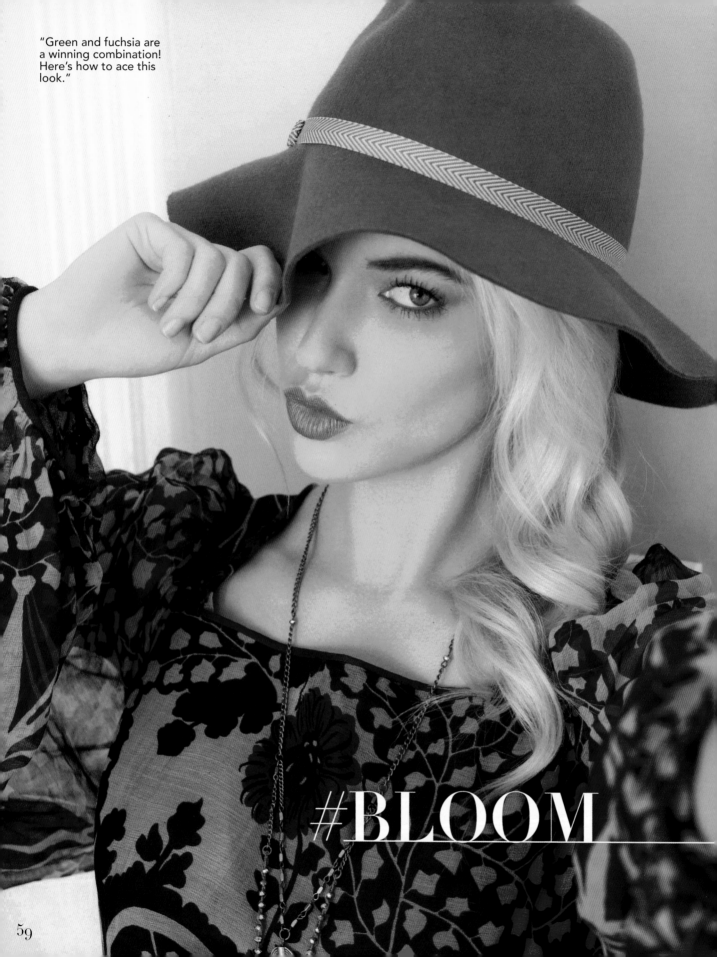

"Green and fuchsia are a winning combination! Here's how to ace this look."

#BLOOM

59

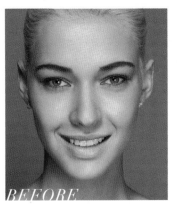

BEFORE

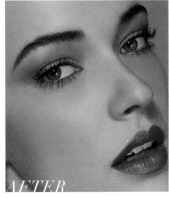

AFTER

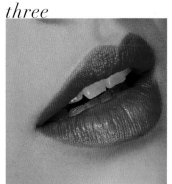

The Essentials

- Concealer
- Translucent powder
- Powder highlighter
- Golden pink blush
- Cheek brush
- Light beige, warm gold and lime-green eye-shadows
- Eyelash curler
- Mascara
- Pink lipstick
- Fuchsia lipstick

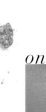

one

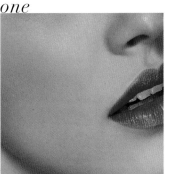

two

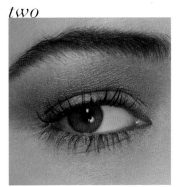

three

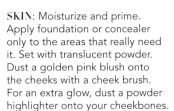

SKIN: Moisturize and prime. Apply foundation or concealer only to the areas that really need it. Set with translucent powder. Dust a golden pink blush onto the cheeks with a cheek brush. For an extra glow, dust a powder highlighter onto your cheekbones.

TIP: *When applying blush, look straight into the mirror and sweep the blush softly onto the apples of the cheeks towards your temple.*

EYES: Dust a warm gold eyeshadow around the eyelid and inner corners. Apply a lime-green eyeshadow onto the lid and blend up to the crease. Curl eyelashes and apply a couple of coats of mascara to both the top and bottom lashes.

TIP: *Powder highlighter can also be dabbed onto the inner corners of the eyes to serve as a brightener!*

LIPS: Exfoliate and moisturize lips, then swipe a soft, velvet-textured pink lipstick and follow with a coat of a fuchsia lipstick. Blot and reapply for a long-lasting application.

TIP: *Layering two coordinating lip colors creates beautiful dimension that photographs really well!*

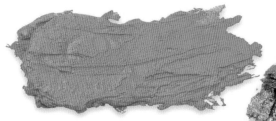

SELFIE TIP:

For the best quality selfie, crop your picture later and don't zoom in while you shoot! While most smartphones have a zoom feature, you will usually get better resolution results by cropping the image later as opposed to zooming in at the start.

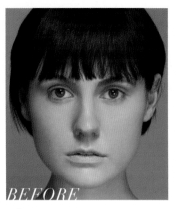
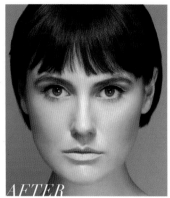

BEFORE *AFTER*

The Essentials

- Light beige and light brown eyeshadows
- Gel or pencil eyeliner in both black and white
- Mascara
- Bronzer
- Coral-pink cheek color
- Creamy pink lipstick

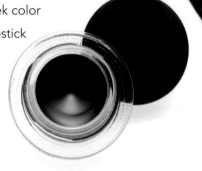

one

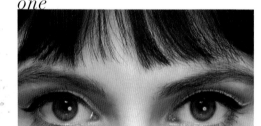

two

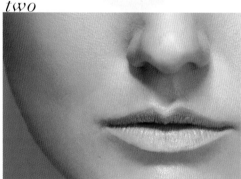

EYES: Apply eye primer to the entire eyelid and lower lash line. Dust a light beige eyeshadow onto the eyelid, then apply a light brown eyeshadow to the crease and the lower lash line to create depth and enlarge the eyes. Starting at the inner corner, draw a thin line with a black gel or pencil eyeliner, creating small lines towards the middle of the eye and elongating and tapering the line towards the outer corner. Repeat the same application with a white gel or pencil eyeliner in white. Apply two coats of mascara to the top and bottom lashes.

TIP: *Hold your eyelid taut with one finger while applying eyeliner.*

CHEEKS & LIPS : Swipe a coral-pink cheek color onto the apples of the cheeks. Use a highlighter to illuminate the tops of the cheeks, the bridge of the nose and the Cupid's bow. Finish the look with a creamy pink lipstick.

TIP: *If you feel that the cheek color looks too strong, dab the area with a clean sponge to remove some of the color. You can also dust a bit of translucent powder on top to tone down the color.*

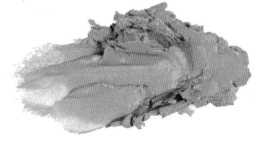

SELFIE TIP:

Use HDR mode. High Dynamic Range is a technology on a smartphone that takes a few pictures at once and combines them into one image. If you are going to be shooting your selfies in an area that has tricky lighting, give HDR a try. And don't worry — your smartphone will usually take both a regular shot and an HDR version for you to choose from later.

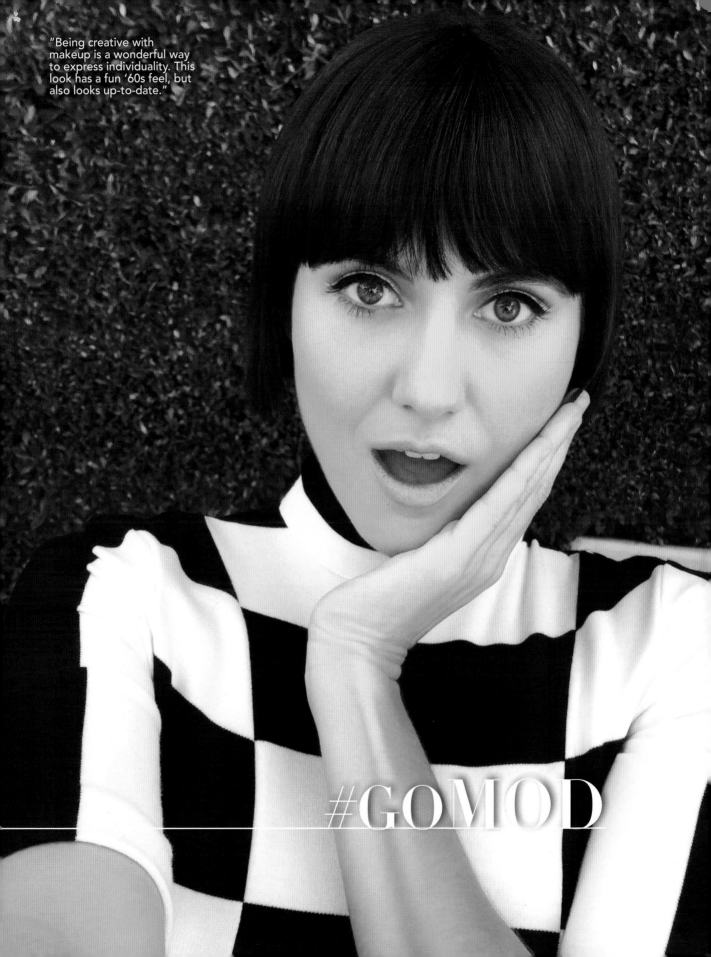

"Being creative with makeup is a wonderful way to express individuality. This look has a fun '60s feel, but also looks up-to-date."

#GOMOD

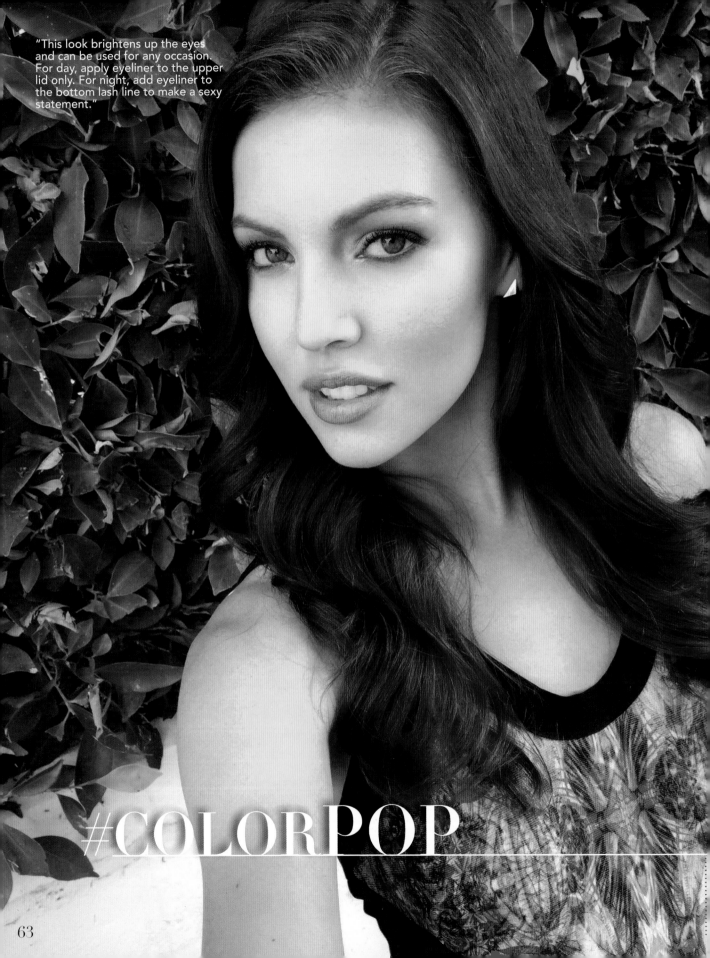

"This look brightens up the eyes and can be used for any occasion. For day, apply eyeliner to the upper lid only. For night, add eyeliner to the bottom lash line to make a sexy statement."

#COLORPOP

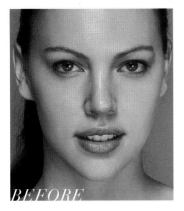
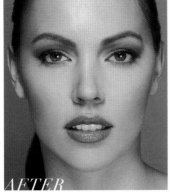

BEFORE *AFTER*

The Essentials

- Light blue cream eyeshadow to serve as a base for the eyeliner
- Light to medium shade of blue powder eyeshadow
- Light brown and pearly gold eyeshadows
- Two angled eyeliner brushes
- Shimmery brown blush
- Neutral lipstick

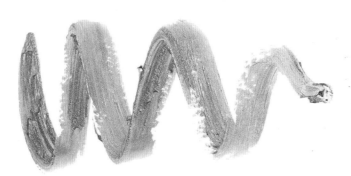
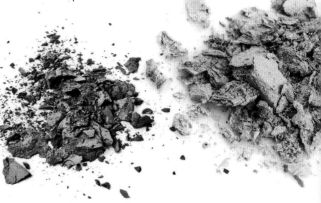

one

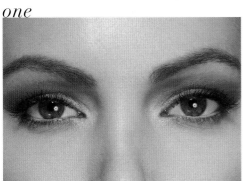

two

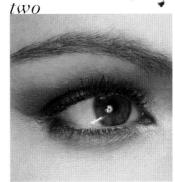

three

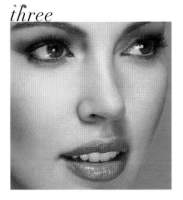

EYES: With a pearly gold eyeshadow, highlight the inner corners of the eye and the eyelid, stopping right under the crease. Add depth at the crease with a light brown eyeshadow and blend well.

EYELINER: At the base of the lashes, use an angled eyeliner brush to swipe a light blue cream eyeshadow around the rims of the eyes. With a clean angled brush, layer on a blue powder eyeshadow. Extend a soft line past the outer corner to create a cat-eye flare.

TIP: *If you don't have a blue cream eyeshadow, dampen a brush and dip it into the powder eyeshadow to create your own cream.*

CHEEKS & LIPS: If you have a long face, apply blush onto the apples of the cheeks and blend the color out towards the ears. Use a shade similar to the eyeshadow used on the crease to create a neutral effect. Use a similar neutral shade for the lips.

TIP: *To make sure your eyeliner pops, keep the rest of the makeup on your face simple and neutral.*

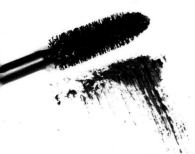
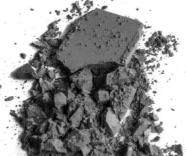

SELFIE TIP:
Use a "burst" effect on your camera when rocking this fun look. Strike a pose and take multiple shots in succession!

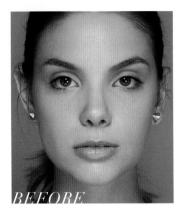

BEFORE

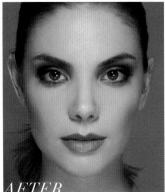

AFTER

The Essentials

- Emerald green, matte purple, soft brown and gold eyeshadows
- Tight bristled synthetic brush
- Fluffy eyeshadow brush
- Angled brush
- Cherry cheek color
- Mascaras in two formulas (regular and water-proof)
- Bronzer
- Bronze-gold lip gloss

one

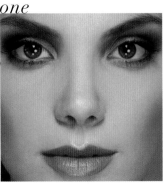

SKIN: Use a foundation brush to apply a thin, even veil of matte foundation to the face, concentrating on the areas that need the most coverage.

TIP: *When blending foundation use small, downward strokes. This will prevent the hairs on your face from standing on end.*

two

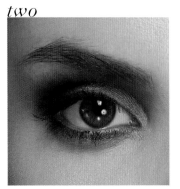

EYES: Prep the eye area with a primer and concealer. Use an eyeshadow brush to pat an emerald green shade from the lash line up to the crease.

TIP: *For precise placement, apply eyeshadow with a tight bristled synthetic brush and pat the shadow onto your eye. Blend with a fluffy eyeshadow brush. Using an angled brush, highlight the inner corners of the eyes with a gold eyeshadow. With a clean brush, apply a matte purple eyeshadow along the lower lash line. Take a brown eyeshadow about two shades darker than your skin tone and blend onto the crease and anywhere else you see hard edges.*

TIP: *You can also use bronzer to smooth out the color on the crease. This is especially useful when blending bright shades!*

three

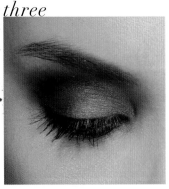

EYELASHES: Try layering two mascaras for maximum impact. Start by curling your lashes and applying either a volumizing or lengthening mascara. Once the mascara is almost dry, follow with a coat of waterproof mascara. If you have a tendency to sweat under your eyes, use only the waterproof mascara on the lower lashes. This combination is great for hard-to-curl lashes and also ensures that any leftover mascara residue will be easy to remove.

four

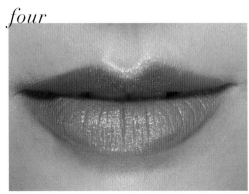

CHEEKS & LIPS: Blend a soft cherry cheek color with a bronzer to create a warm, natural-looking shade. Finish with a sheer bronze-gold lip gloss.

TIP: *Your eyes shouldn't compete with your lips, so when wearing a dramatic eye, go with a neutral shade lip!*

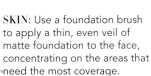
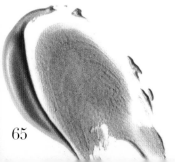

SELFIE TIP:
Love your selfie but can't get rid of the glare of the light? Try cupping your hand over the lens when taking your picture to cut down the amount of glare — it works!

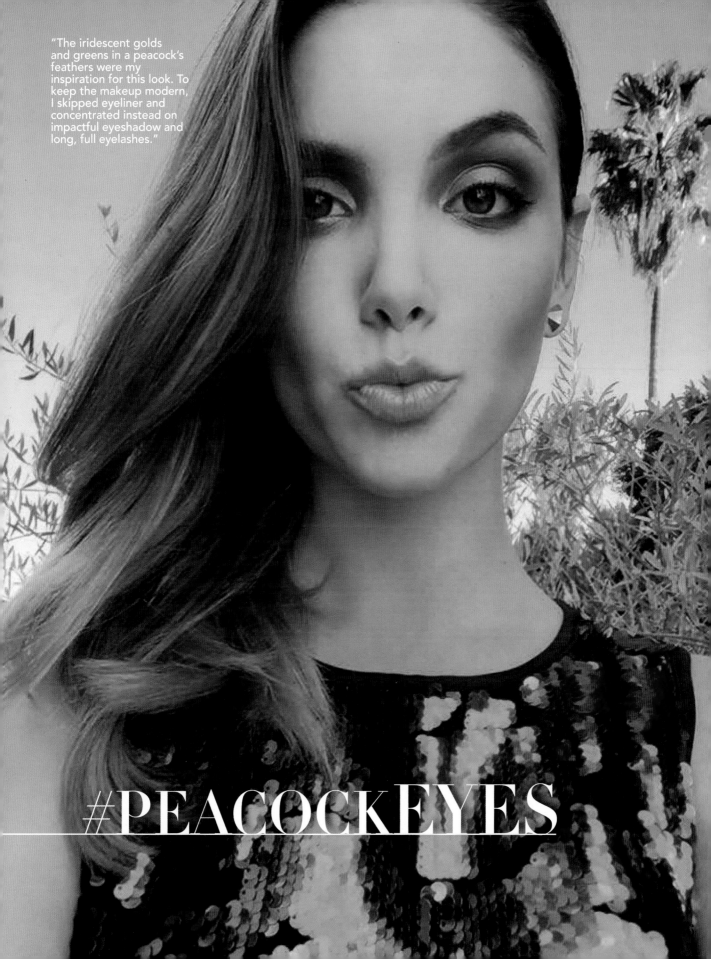

"The iridescent golds and greens in a peacock's feathers were my inspiration for this look. To keep the makeup modern, I skipped eyeliner and concentrated instead on impactful eyeshadow and long, full eyelashes."

#PEACOCKEYES

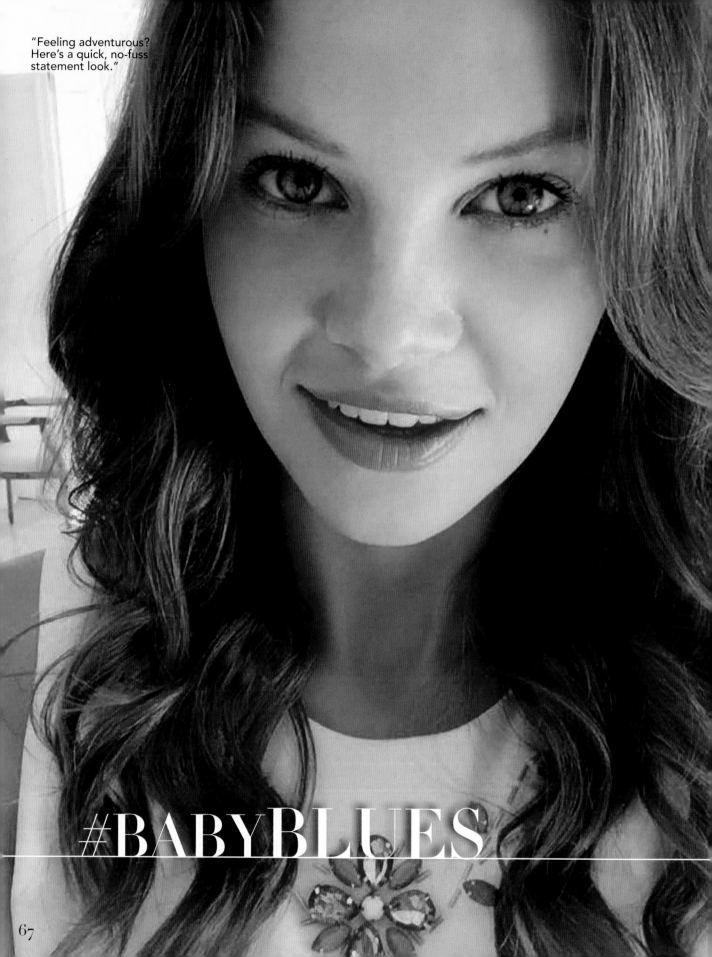

"Feeling adventurous? Here's a quick, no-fuss statement look."

#BABYBLUES

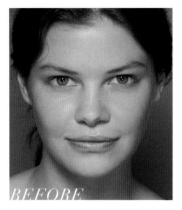
BEFORE

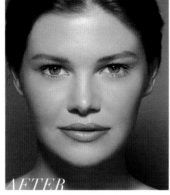
AFTER

The Essentials

- Tinted moisturizer (or BB or CC cream) with SPF
- Mascara
- Blue crayon eyeshadow
- Silver powder eyeshadow
- Light peach cheek color
- Rose tinted lip balm

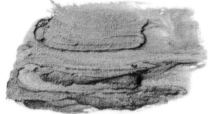

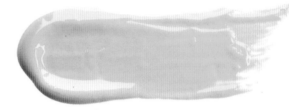

one

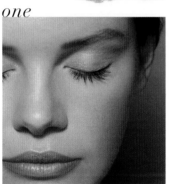

two

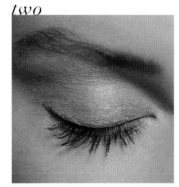

three

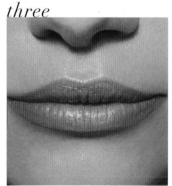

SKIN: Dot the forehead, tip of nose, chin and cheeks with a tinted moisturizer, BB or CC cream with SPF. Blend well. Sun damage is no joke and you need to protect your skin no matter what your age. Make sure your coverage cream has SPF!

TIP: *For light coverage and extra SPF protection, mix sunscreen with a CC cream in the palm of your hands, then apply.*

EYES: Use a teal blue eyeliner crayon or chubby pencil to draw a thick line along the upper lash line. Use your fingers to blend. Repeat as needed, carrying the color up to the eyelid as desired. Dab a light silver shadow over the blue, starting at the base of the lashes. Blend well and follow with two coats of mascara.

TIP: *This technique works well with any shade — the pencil's waxy texture makes it easy to blend.*

CHEEKS & LIPS: Dust a light peach blush onto the apples of the cheeks and blend. Finish the look with a creamy pink lipstick and a pink lip gloss on top, if desired.

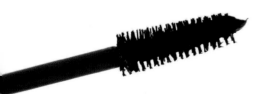

SELFIE TIP:
When shooting inside, remember that the light can change from room to room. Don't be afraid to walk around and find the best possible light in which to snap your selfie.

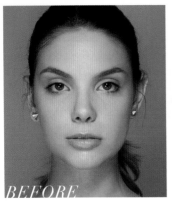

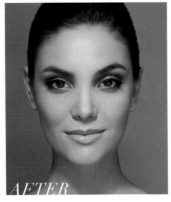

BEFORE   AFTER

The Essentials

- Warm gold and matte brown eyeshadows
- Black gel eyeliner
- Mascara
- Golden pink cheek color
- Bronzer
- Powder brush
- Lip exfoliator and balm
- Neutral lip liner and lipstick

one

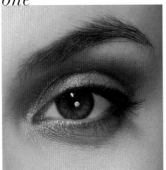

two

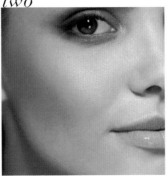

three

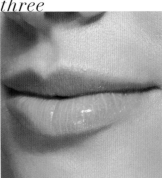

EYES: Start by applying a warm gold eye color to the lid, stopping at the crease. Dab the same shade onto the lower lash line, concentrating on the inner corners. Next, sweep a matte brown eye color onto the crease, the outer "V" and the outer three-fourths of the bottom lash line. Blend thoroughly. Line the upper lash line with a black gel eyeliner, starting with a very thin line at the inner corners that thickens as it reaches the outer corners. Finish with two coats of lengthening mascara.

TIP: Matte eyeshadows are often difficult to blend, so use a clean blending brush and make back-and-forth windshield wiper motions to blend out any hard edges

CHEEKS: Give the skin a bronzy glow by using a bronzer and cheek color combination. Apply a warm, golden pink blush to the cheeks, then apply bronzer wherever the sun would natural hit your face (such as the tops of cheeks and the temples). With a clean powder brush, blend the blush and bronzer together for a smooth, glowing effect.

LIPS: Exfoliate the lips and follow with balm. Dab a small amount of foundation onto your lips if you have any discoloration. Apply a neutral lip liner all over the lips and finish off with a neutral shade of lipstick.

TIP: For a natural-looking nude effect, try using a lip liner and lipstick that are the same shade and just slightly darker than your natural lip color.

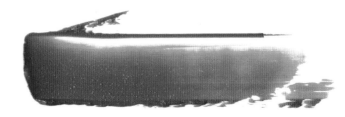

SELFIE TIP:

There's nothing wrong with using a filter to brighten up a self-ie on a gloomy day!

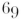

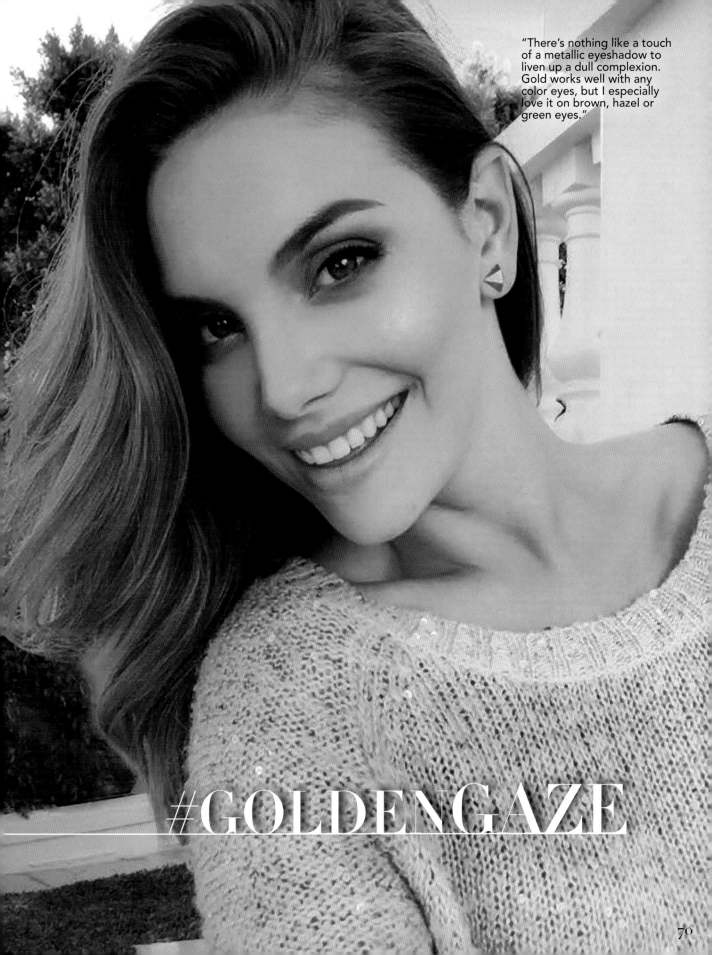

"There's nothing like a touch of a metallic eyeshadow to liven up a dull complexion. Gold works well with any color eyes, but I especially love it on brown, hazel or green eyes."

#GOLDENGAZE

"This technique gives your eyes an instant lift. I used a soft plum shade here, but don't be afraid to make your own statement and try other colors!"

#SPARKLINGPLUM

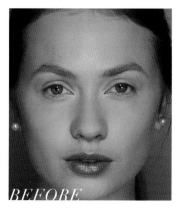

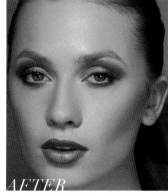

BEFORE *AFTER*

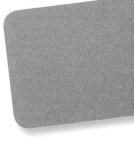

The Essentials

- Eyebrow pencil
- Eyebrow gel
- Silver and light plum eyeshadows
- Flat eyeshadow brush
- Mascara
- Soft berry blush
- Light mauve lipstick

one

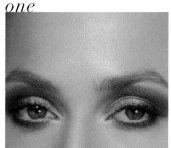

two

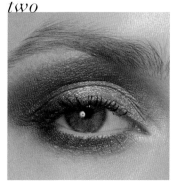

three

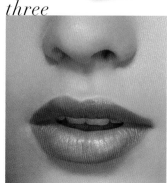

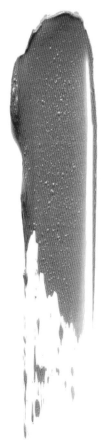

EYEBROWS: Keep the focus on the eyes by using an eyebrow pencil that's slightly lighter than the color of your natural brows. Starting at your brow's arch, fill in sparse areas with short strokes. Follow with an eyebrow gel to set.

TIP: *Leave the inner corners alone for a groomed yet natural look.*

EYES: Apply a lustrous silver eyeshadow from the inner corner to the middle of the lid. Using a flat eyeliner brush, create a thick, cat-eye-esque line with a light violet eyeshadow at the outer corner, bringing it into the crease area and along lower lash line. Blend well using another clean eyeshadow brush. Curl the eyelashes and add a couple of coats of mascara on both the top and bottom lashes.

CHEEKS & LIPS: Dust a soft berry blush on the hollows of the cheeks, blending up to the temples. Use a clean powder brush to blend into a soft hue. With your fingertips, tap a light mauve lipstick onto the middle of the lips, then spread the color evenly for a natural stain.

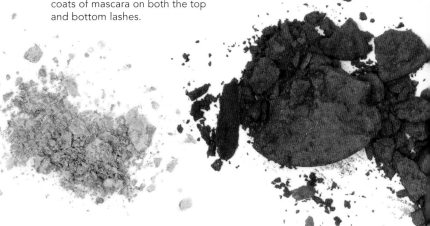

SELFIE TIP:

North- and south-facing windows will usually give you the best light, depending on the time of day. Just remember that the bigger the window, the more light you'll get!

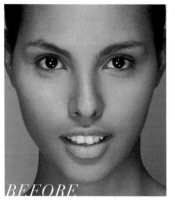

BEFORE

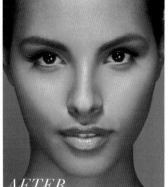

AFTER

The Essentials

- Foundation
- Darker matte powder or bronzer
- Peachy pink blush
- Matte off-white and brown eyeshadows
- Eyeshadow brush
- Cheek brush, powder brush, and crease brush
- Liquid or gel eyeliner
- Mascara
- Nude lip liner
- Nude brown lipstick

one

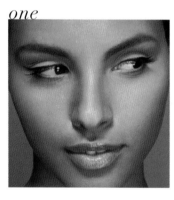

two

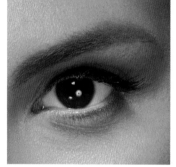

three

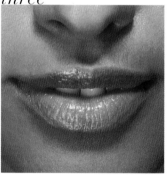

SKIN: Apply foundation to clean, moisturized skin. Use a cheek brush and a dark matte powder to contour the hollows of the cheeks, the temples, the nose and under the jawline. Use a powder brush to blend, and dust on a little translucent powder to smooth any harsh lines.

TIP: *The trick to good contouring is to use the product that works best for you (either foundation, concealer or powder) and to blend it thoroughly, until it's virtually undetectable.*

EYES: With an eyeshadow brush, tap an off-white matte shadow all over the eyelid. Sculpt the crease and the lower lash line with a matte brown eyeshadow. Use a clean crease brush to blend. You can also use a brown eyeliner to create the same effect by lining around the crease and lower lash line and blending with a brush. Follow by applying liquid eyeliner along the top lash lines only, thickening the line as desired. Finish with a coat of mascara.

TIP: *Enhance the eye area by adding a few fake eyelashes at the corner of the eyes. Apply one coat of mascara first, then add the lashes. Once they're dry, apply one more coat of mascara to blend the faux lashes with your own.*

CHEEKS & LIPS: Dust a peachy pink blush onto the apples of the cheeks and blend into the bronzer. Finish off by dusting a highlighter over the blush and onto bridge of the nose and Cupid's bow. Line the lips with a neutral lip liner and fill in with a nude shade of creamy lipstick. Blot and reapply.

SELFIE TIP:

Keep your hand steady! It's simply the best way to avoid blurry selfies. If possible, try to rest your arm on a wall or place your elbow on a steady surface while taking your selfie.

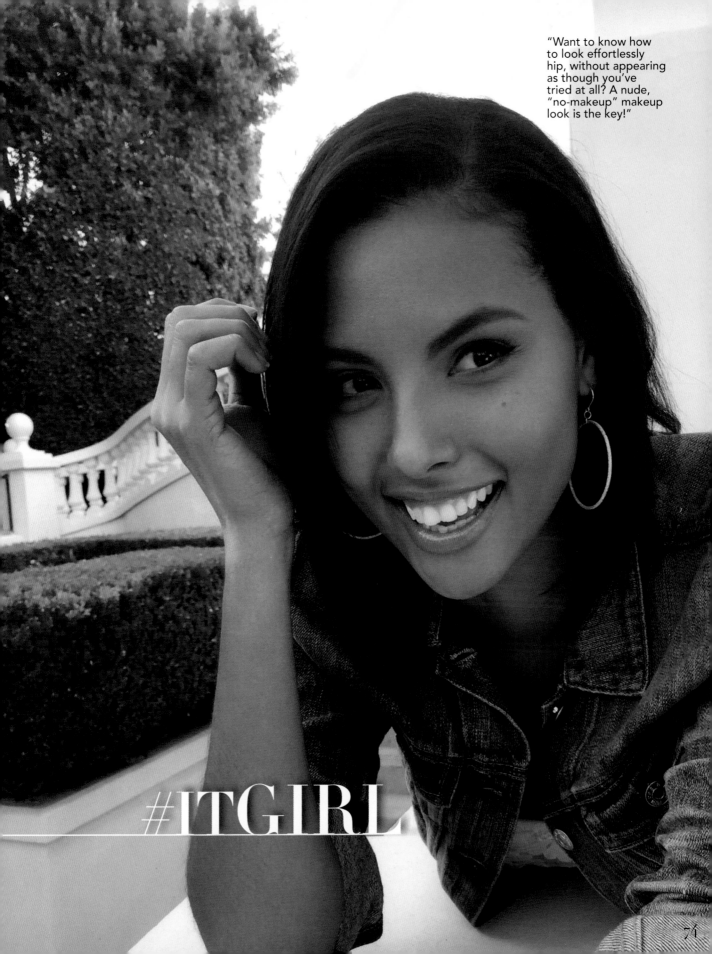

"Want to know how to look effortlessly hip, without appearing as though you've tried at all? A nude, "no-makeup" makeup look is the key!"

#ITGIRL

71

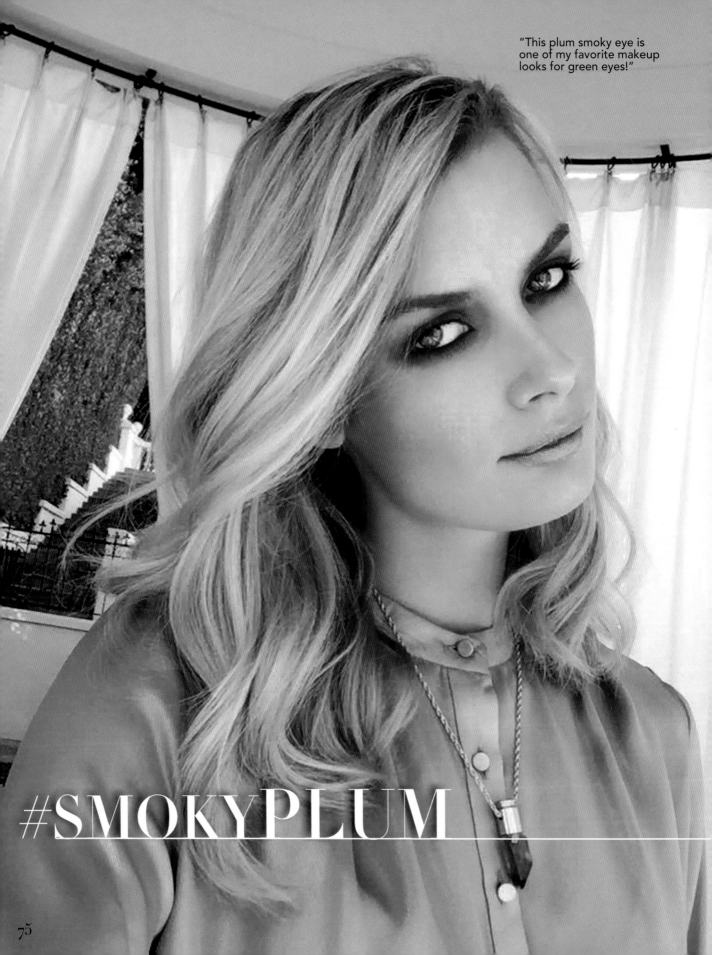

"This plum smoky eye is one of my favorite makeup looks for green eyes!"

#SMOKYPLUM

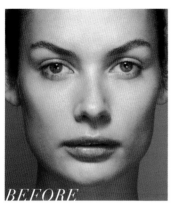

BEFORE

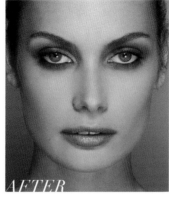

AFTER

The Essentials

- Eyebrow pencil
- Eyebrow gel
- Eyelash primer
- Black pencil eyeliner
- Plum and soft purple eyeshadows
- Peachy pink blush
- Eyelash curler
- Mascara

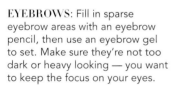

one

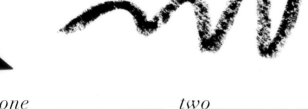

two

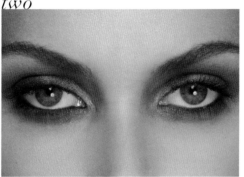

three

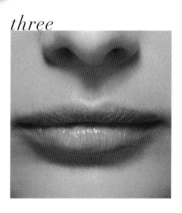

EYEBROWS: Fill in sparse eyebrow areas with an eyebrow pencil, then use an eyebrow gel to set. Make sure they're not too dark or heavy looking — you want to keep the focus on your eyes.

TIP: *A smoky eye always looks best with nicely groomed brows.*

EYES: Dab an eye primer over the entire eyelid and along the lower lash line. Primer makes eyeshadow easier to apply and will keep color from creasing or fading. Using an eyeshadow brush, dust a light plum eyeshadow all around the eyes, right up to the crease. Starting at the outer corners, shade the crease and the lower lash line with a soft purple or violet shadow. Use a clean crease brush to soften all edges. If desired, create a line very close to the waterline with a black eyeliner pencil or gel.

EYELASHES: Curl clean eyelashes with an eyelash curler to give them lift. Follow with a coat of either a lengthening or a volumizing mascara.

TIP: *If you have thin eyelashes, coat them with an eyelash primer before you apply your mascara.*

CHEEKS & LIPS: Dust a slightly shimmery, peachy pink shade of blush onto your cheeks. Pair it with a natural, sheer gloss.

SELFIE TIP:

For the best quality pictures shoot your selfie with your phone's display facing away from you, so that you're looking directly into the lens. Can't stand not seeing what you look like? Try taking your selfie in front of a mirror.

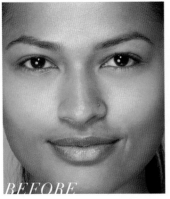
BEFORE

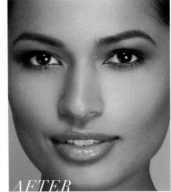
AFTER

The Essentials

- Sparkling blue and matte brown eyeshadows
- Small eyeshadow brush
- Synthetic eyeshadow brush
- Black gel eyeliner
- Golden peach blush
- Nude lipstick

one

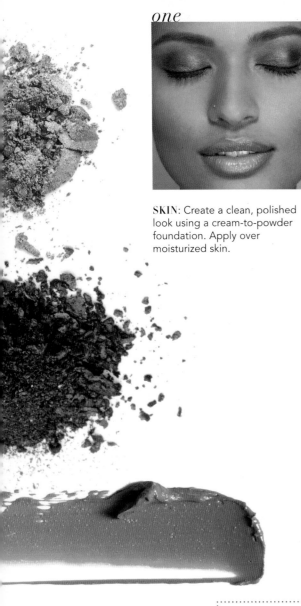

two

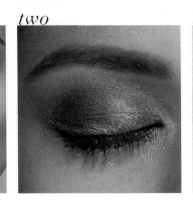

three

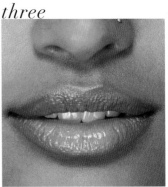

SKIN: Create a clean, polished look using a cream-to-powder foundation. Apply over moisturized skin.

EYES: Pat an eye primer or blue eyeshadow crayon onto the eyelid with either your fingertips or a small synthetic brush. Sweep dark blue eyeshadow on top and along the lower lash line. Be sure to make this line narrow and thin so your eyes don't look droopy.

TIP: *Scared of bright blue? Try a darker shade, like navy. The darker the hue, the more wearable the blue color becomes. Dust a matte brown eyeshadow at the crease, blending away any hard edges created by the blue shadow. With an angled brush, line the base of the upper lash line with a black gel eyeliner. Finish by curling your lashes and applying two to three coats of mascara.*

TIP: *When attempting a smoky eye, apply concealer after you are done with the eyes. This allows you to clean up any smears or smudges and correct the eyeshadow shape, if necessary.*

CHEEKS & LIPS: Blend a golden peach blush into the cheeks. Line the lips fully to combat any discoloration and follow with a natural, earth-toned lipstick.

SELFIE TIP:
Don't ignore your eyebrows! Perfectly groomed brows will make your selfie look amazing.

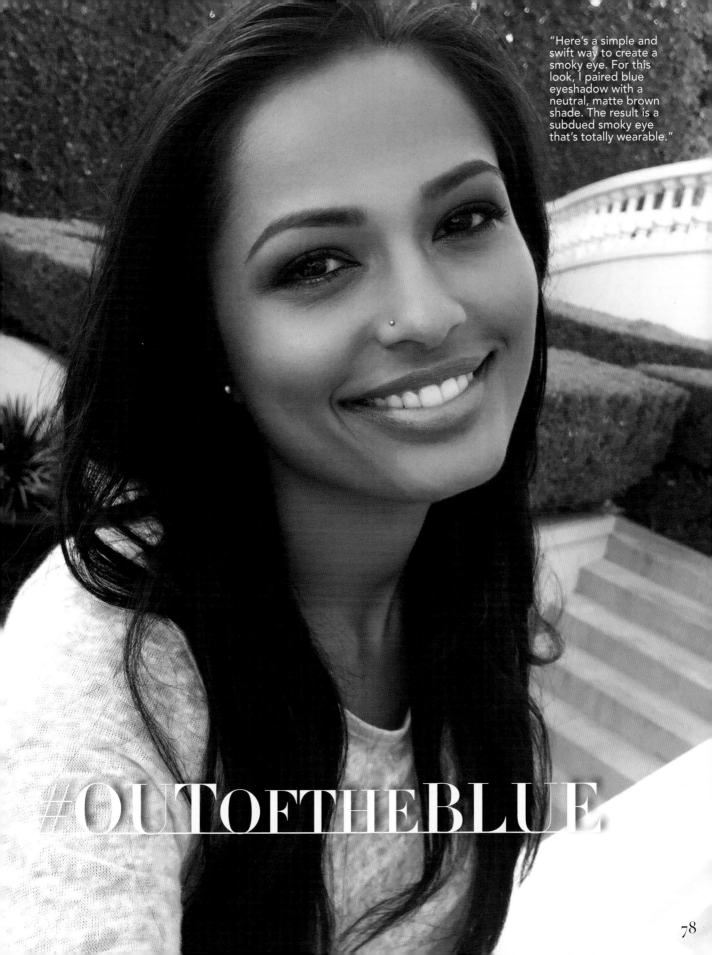

"Here's a simple and swift way to create a smoky eye. For this look, I paired blue eyeshadow with a neutral, matte brown shade. The result is a subdued smoky eye that's totally wearable."

#OUTOFTHEBLUE

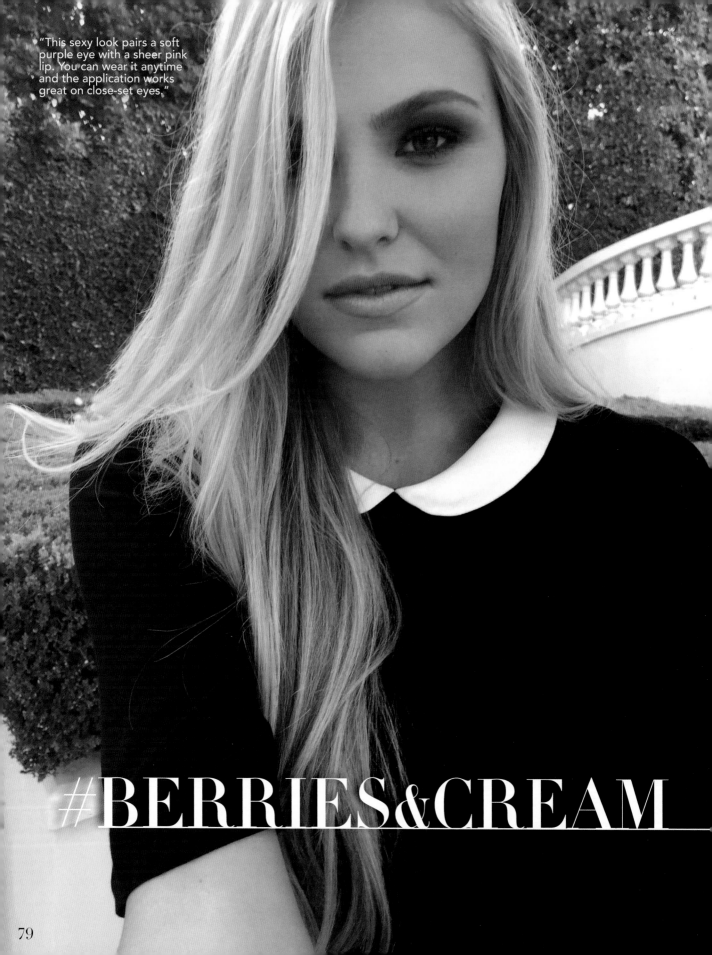

"This sexy look pairs a soft purple eye with a sheer pink lip. You can wear it anytime and the application works great on close-set eyes."

#BERRIES&CREAM

79

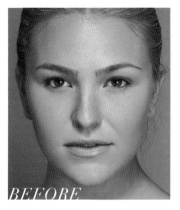
BEFORE

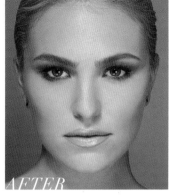
AFTER

The Essentials

- Light lavender and dark lavender eyeshadows
- Translucent powder
- Flat eyeshadow brush
- Fluffy blending brush
- Mascara
- Pearly pink cheek color
- Sheer pink lipstick

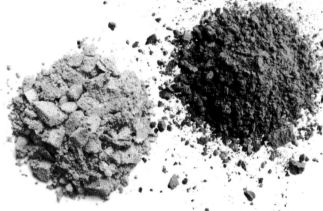

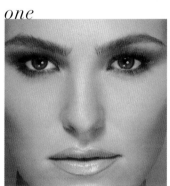

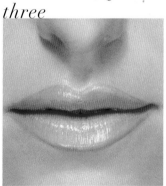

one

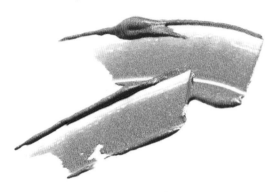

two

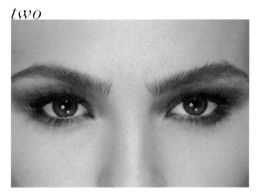

three

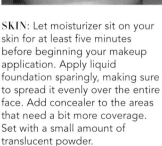

SKIN: Let moisturizer sit on your skin for at least five minutes before beginning your makeup application. Apply liquid foundation sparingly, making sure to spread it evenly over the entire face. Add concealer to the areas that need a bit more coverage. Set with a small amount of translucent powder.

EYES: Apply eyeshadow primer to the eyelid and bottom lash line. With a flat eyeshadow brush, tap a light lavender eyeshadow from lid to crease, starting at the outer corners. Blend from the lash line up to the crease. Next, shade the crease and the lower lash line with a slightly darker violet shade. Use a large, clean brush to blend upwards, towards the brow bone and the outer third of the top eyelid. Softly line the upper lash line with a black eyeliner pencil to intensify the look and blend with a smudger brush to soften. Apply two coats of mascara to both the top and bottom lashes.

LIPS: Dust the apples of the cheeks with a soft pink blush to create a natural-looking flush. Follow with a sheer pink lipstick.

SELFIE TIP:

Can't seem to find good lighting? Bring the camera closer to your face. You'll have more control over your shot and will be better able to block out any unflattering light so your selfie looks #onpoint!

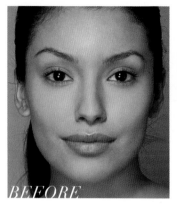

BEFORE

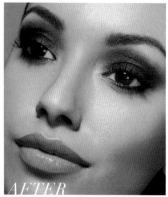

AFTER

The Essentials

- Matte coverage foundation
- Loose powder
- Powder puff and powder brush
- Black, copper-brown and shimmery deep blue eyeshadows
- Tapered eyeshadow brush
- Black gel or liquid eyeliner
- Black mascara
- Warm copper blush
- Nude lipstick

one

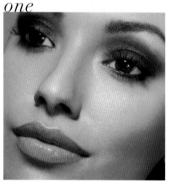

two

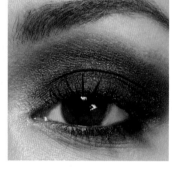

EYES: Smooth eye primer over the eyelids. With a tapered eyeshadow brush, tap a slightly shimmery deep blue eyeshadow onto the eyelids. Shade up to the crease, the inner corners and along the lower lash line. Blend a copper-brown eyeshadow at the crease and along the lower third of the eye. Starting at the outer corners, use a smudger brush to line the eyes with a black eyeshadow, then soften the line and blend up to create a smoky effect. Finish by applying two coats of mascara to the top and bottom lashes.

TIP: *Larger eyes can handle smoky shades that blend past the crease, while smaller hooded eyes look better with a less intense smoky look that stays close to the lash line.*

EYELINER: To deepen the look, use a gel or liquid eyeliner on the top lash line and blend into the black shadow.

SKIN: A look like this calls for skin that looks flawless. Use a primer and follow with a matte foundation. Set with loose powder where needed.

TIP: *Like a matte look? Use a powder puff to apply loose powder and concentrate on the T-zone area. Buff away excess powder with a clean powder puff.*

three

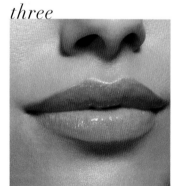

CHEEKS & LIPS: Keep the focus on the eyes by applying a warm bronze blush and a nude lipstick.

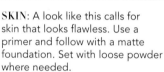

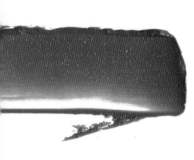

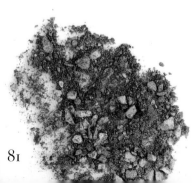

SELFIE TIP:

Find the right light! A deep, sultry eye like this one looks best when light shines directly in front of your face. Avoid any unwanted shadows.

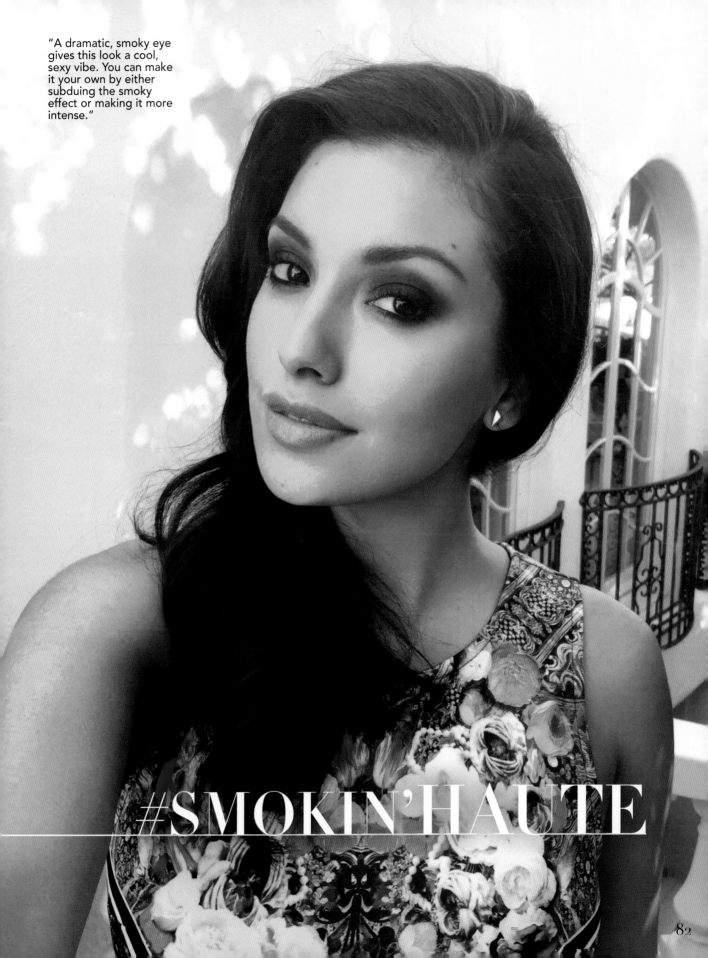

"A dramatic, smoky eye gives this look a cool, sexy vibe. You can make it your own by either subduing the smoky effect or making it more intense."

#SMOKIN'HAUTE

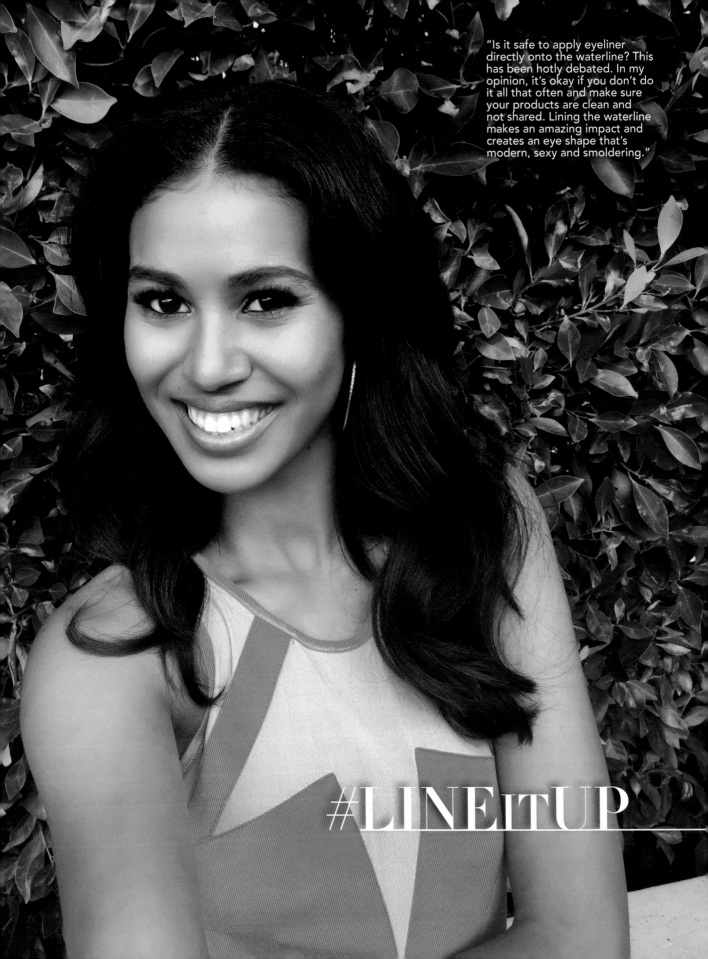

"Is it safe to apply eyeliner directly onto the waterline? This has been hotly debated. In my opinion, it's okay if you don't do it all that often and make sure your products are clean and not shared. Lining the waterline makes an amazing impact and creates an eye shape that's modern, sexy and smoldering."

#LINEitUP

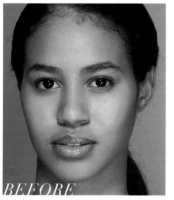

BEFORE

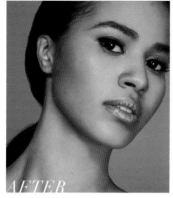

AFTER

The Essentials

- Warm gold, light bone and soft brown eyeshadows
- Black gel eyeliner
- Eyeliner brush
- Individual false eyelashes
- Mascara
- Bronzer
- Nude lipstick

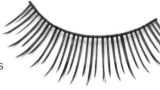

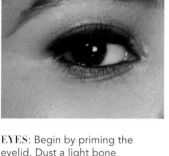

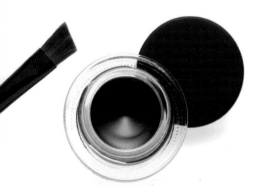

one

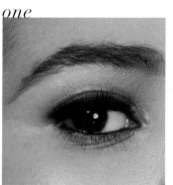

two

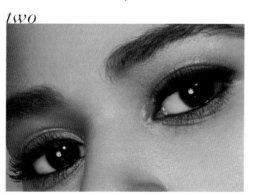

three

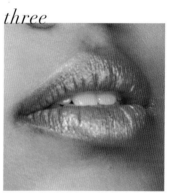

EYES: Begin by priming the eyelid. Dust a light bone eyeshadow onto the lid from lash line to brow, then apply a slightly sparkly warm gold eyeshadow onto the lid and inner corners. Follow by adding a warm brown shade at the outer corners and on the crease. Blend well.

EYELINER: Pull the eye taut and trace small strokes inside the lower waterline with a gel eyeliner and brush. Blink a couple of times to even the distribution. Using another eyeliner brush, line the upper lashes, getting as close to the base as possible. Keep the line thin and elongated at the outer corner for a winged effect. Apply faux lashes if desired and finish off with mascara.

TIP: *Don't forget to let the lash glue dry for a few seconds before you apply fake lashes. Increase the cat-eye effect by adding a little lift to the lashes at the outer corners of the eyes.*

CHEEKS & LIPS: With an intense eye look like this one, it's best to keep the rest of your makeup natural. Use a bronzer to sculpt the face along the hollows of the cheeks, the sides of the nose and underneath the chin. Dust on a warm bronze brush, then finish off the look with a creamy beige lipstick.

SELFIE TIP:

Get a reflector! Sometimes a little bounce of light can really make a difference. You can buy one at a camera store, or you can simply place a white piece of cardboard in front or under your face. Ask any photographer — they all use them!

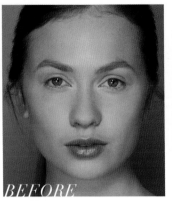
BEFORE

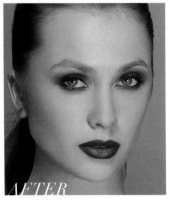
AFTER

The Essentials

- Light eyebrow pencil or matte eyeshadow
- Eyebrow gel
- Plum eyeshadow
- Makeup sponge
- Black gel or pencil eyeliner
- Berry or plum shade of cheek and lip tint
- Lip liner

one

two

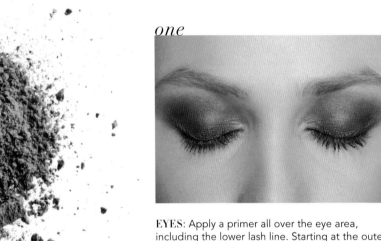

EYES: Apply a primer all over the eye area, including the lower lash line. Starting at the outer corners, use a plum eyeshadow to encircle the eye with a light wash of color. Blend the edges well. Line the base of both the upper and lower lashes with a gel eyeliner.

EYEBROWS: Lightly fill the brows with a pencil or eyeshadow. Sweep the hairs up, out and towards the temples with an eyebrow gel to set the hairs in place.

CHEEKS & LIPS: Smile and add a couple of dots of a berry cream blush onto the apples of your cheeks. Blend with a sponge.

TIP: *If the cheek color looks too dark, blend in a little foundation to tone down the hue. Use the same product over the lips and follow with a lip liner, if needed..*

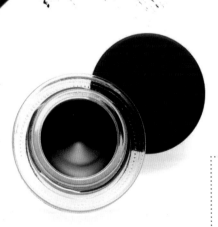

SELFIE TIP:
When taking a selfie with heavily made-up eyes and lips, make sure your light is soft and indirect. Harsh light can make the look appear overdone.

#BERRYDEEP

86

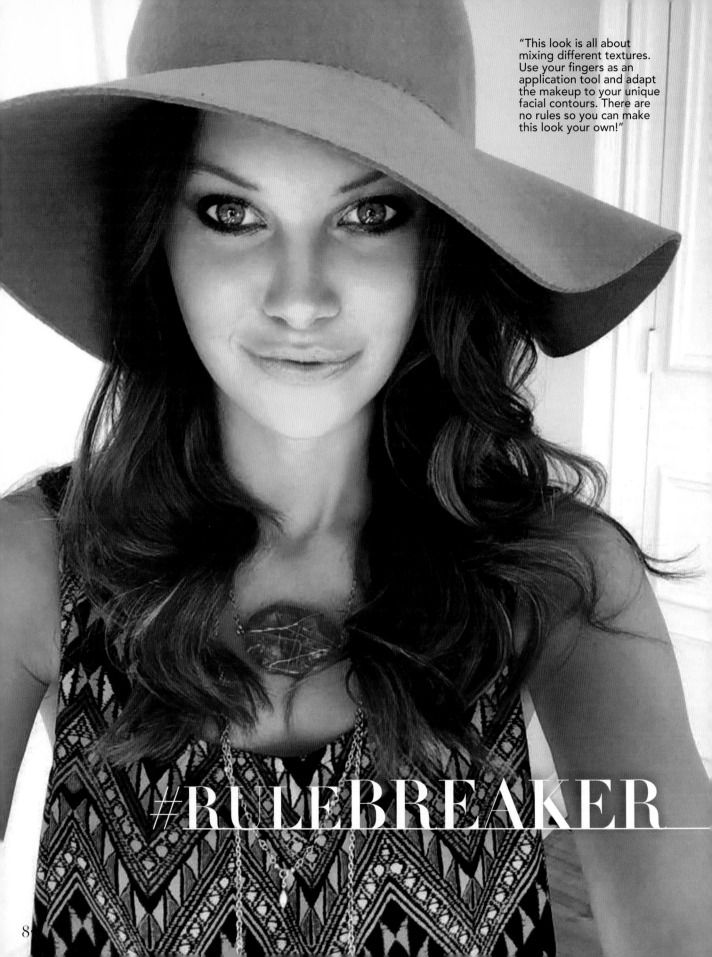

"This look is all about mixing different textures. Use your fingers as an application tool and adapt the makeup to your unique facial contours. There are no rules so you can make this look your own!"

#RULEBREAKER

8

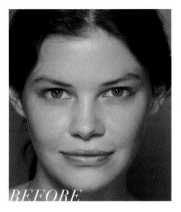

BEFORE

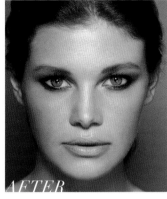

AFTER

The Essentials

- Foundation or CC cream
- Creamy silver, powder silver and black eyeshadows
- Eyelash curler
- Lash primer
- Mascara
- Natural cheek color
- Lipstick

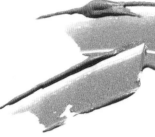

one

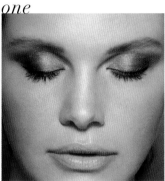

two

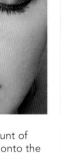

three

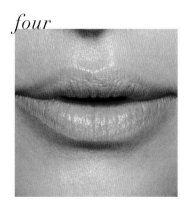

SKIN: Place a small amount of foundation or CC cream onto the back of your hand, then use a brush or your fingertips to blend it into your face until it disappears into your skin. Use light layers and concentrate on areas that need the most coverage. Follow with concealer, if needed.

EYES: With your eyes closed, use your finger to pat a cream silver eyeshadow onto the lid. Blend the eyeshadow from the lash line to just above the crease, as well as along the lower lash line. With a clean brush, blend a silver powder eyeshadow on top. Smudge a black or dark gray eyeshadow at the upper and lower lash lines to create depth. If you'd like, extend the line into an outer V to deepen the look.

EYELASHES: This look is all about the lashes! Begin by curling the lashes and applying a lash primer to fortify and add volume. For a long and lifted look, apply mascara onto the tips of your lashes first, then move the wand from the roots up.

TIP: *Holding the mascara wand for a few seconds at the tip of freshly curled lashes creates a long-lasting curl.*

four

CHEEKS & LIPS: Apply a rosy cheek color that is similar in shade to your natural flush. Pair it with a similar natural shade on your lips.

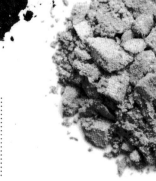

SELFIE TIP:
Become your own fashion stylist and coordinate your outfit with your makeup and hair.

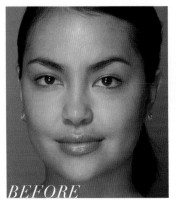

BEFORE

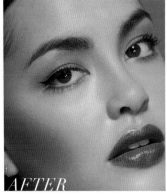

AFTER

The Essentials

- Mineral powder foundation
- Concealer one shade lighter than your skin tone
- Warm pink eyeshadow
- Eyeshadow, cheek and powder brushes
- Liquid eyeliner
- Mascara
- Bronzer
- Caramel-brown lipstick

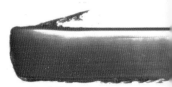

one

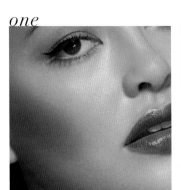

two

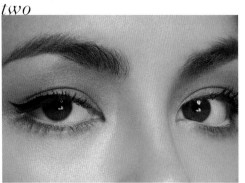

three

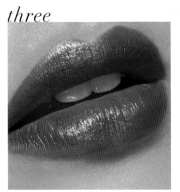

SKIN: Start by moisturizing and priming the skin, then smooth on your choice of foundation. A mineral powder foundation works well for this look because it provides light coverage and gives the skin a smooth and natural finish.

EYES: Apply a concealer that's one shade lighter than your skin tone to your eyelids and blend. With a fluffy eyeshadow brush, lightly pat a warm pink eyeshadow onto your lid and blend up to the crease. Pull your eye slightly taught and draw a thin line along the lash line with a liquid eyeliner pen. Elongate the eye by extending it out in a flick at the outer corners. Follow with two coats of mascara.

TIP: *When wearing a pink eyeshadow, it's best to neutralize any pink and red tones around eyes with concealer. You can also use eye drops, if necessary.*

CHEEKS & LIPS: If you have a round face, use a cheek brush to dust bronzer in an "E" shape at the sides of the face. Then take a bigger powder brush and blend. Swipe a rich and creamy caramel-brown color on your lips.

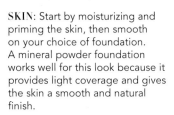
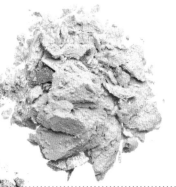
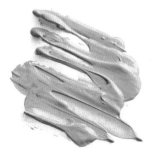
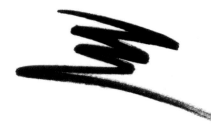

SELFIE TIP:

When taking a really close-up selfie try using a creamy, textured lipstick or gloss and even an eyeshadow with a little shimmer. These products seem to disappear into the skin and create a soft texture that looks #beautiful up close.

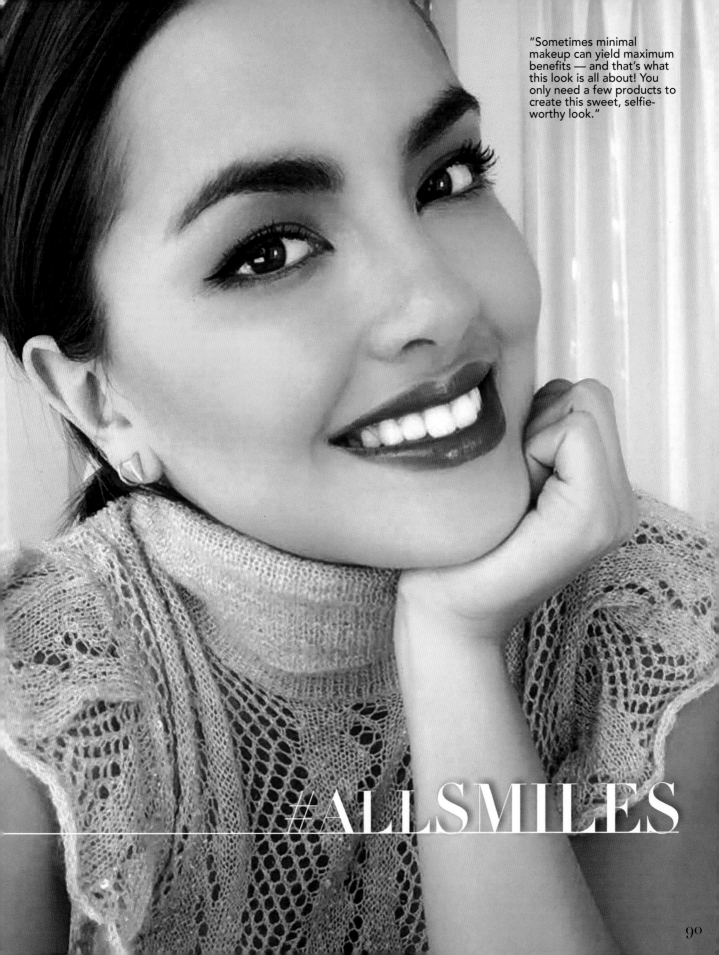

"Sometimes minimal makeup can yield maximum benefits — and that's what this look is all about! You only need a few products to create this sweet, selfie-worthy look."

#ALLSMILES

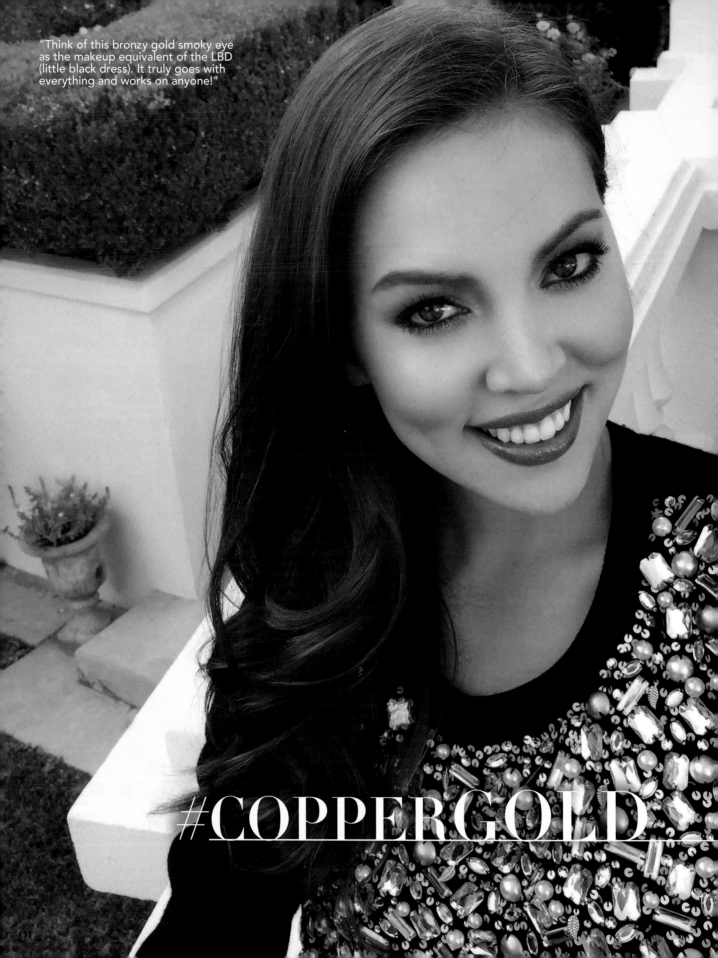

"Think of this bronzy gold smoky eye as the makeup equivalent of the LBD (little black dress). It truly goes with everything and works on anyone!"

#COPPERGOLD

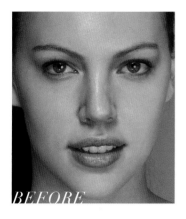
BEFORE

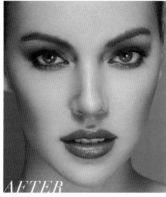
AFTER

The Essentials

- Light iridescent, brown iridescent and copper cream eyeshadows
- Black gel or pencil eyeliner
- Peachy brown cream blush
- Mascara
- Bronzer at least one shade darker than your skin tone
- Copper, gold or brown lipstick
- Gold lip gloss

one

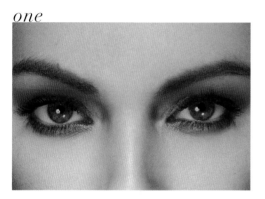

two

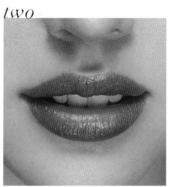

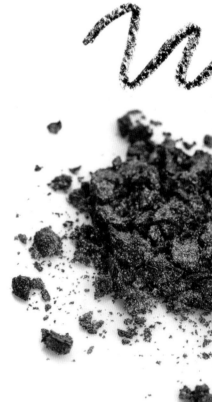

EYES: Apply a copper cream eyeshadow or eye crayon from the lash line to the brow bone. Smudge the same shade along the bottom lash line, just below the eye. "Tightline" the top and bottom lash lines with a black gel or pencil eyeliner. Use a brush to lightly smudge the line into the copper shade. Use an iridescent brown eyeshadow to smudge the black liner up towards the crease. On the lower lash line, blend a gold eyeshadow into the eyeliner for a slight metallic sparkle. Pat a light, iridescent eyeshadow into the inner corners of the eyes for a brightening effect. Follow with mascara on the top and bottom lashes.

TIP: *When smudging a gel eyeliner, blend quickly right after you apply.*

CHEEKS & LIPS: Define the cheeks with a peachy brown cream blush and top with a powder bronzer. This texture combination is my favorite way to give the whole face a sun-kissed look. Fill the lips with a neutral lip liner to correct any imperfections. Top it off with a brown lipstick. Finish with a gold lip gloss applied just to the center of the lips.

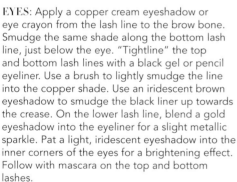

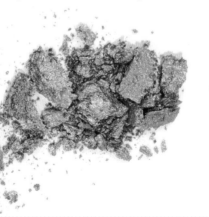

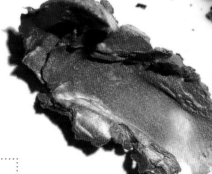

SELFIE TIP:
Go ahead and ham it up! There's nothing wrong with a selfie that shows a wide range of emotion.

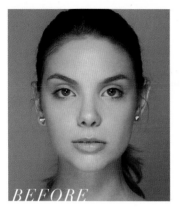
BEFORE

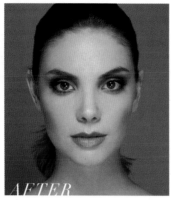
AFTER

The Essentials

- Makeup finishing spray
- Emerald-green and black eyeshadows
- Mascara
- Two fluffy eyeshadow brushes, a blending brush, an angled eyeliner brush and a cheek/bronzer brush
- Nude or very natural shade of lipstick
- Neutral cheek color
- Bronzer
- Sheer nude lipstick

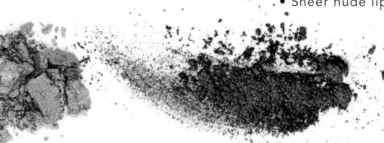

one

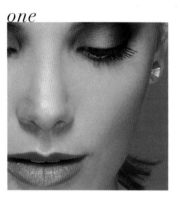

two

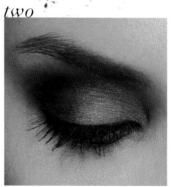

three

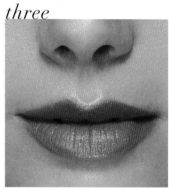

SKIN: Dust on some more translucent powder to reduce shine. Set the look with few pumps of a makeup finishing spray over the face. It will keep your makeup looking fresh it for hours!

EYES: With an eyeshadow brush, apply a warm green eyeshadow over the #goldengaze look on the lid, starting at the outer corners and moving under the lower lash line. To create the smoky effect, use a black or charcoal eyeshadow to intensify the eyeliner and blend into the emerald-green shade. With a clean brush, blend all edges for a seamless look. Finish off with another coat of mascara.

CHEEKS AND LIPS: It's best to use a very neutral palette on the cheeks and lips when wearing a smoky eye. Use a cheek brush and bronzer to further sculpt the hollows of the cheeks, chin and temples, blending any edges with a larger powder brush. Follow with another coat of a sheer nude lipstick.

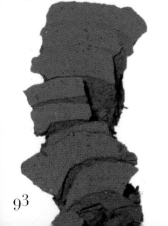

SELFIE TIP:
Want your neck to look longer in your selfies? Bring your forehead slightly forward and down when you take your picture. This will emphasize your jawline and elongate your neck.

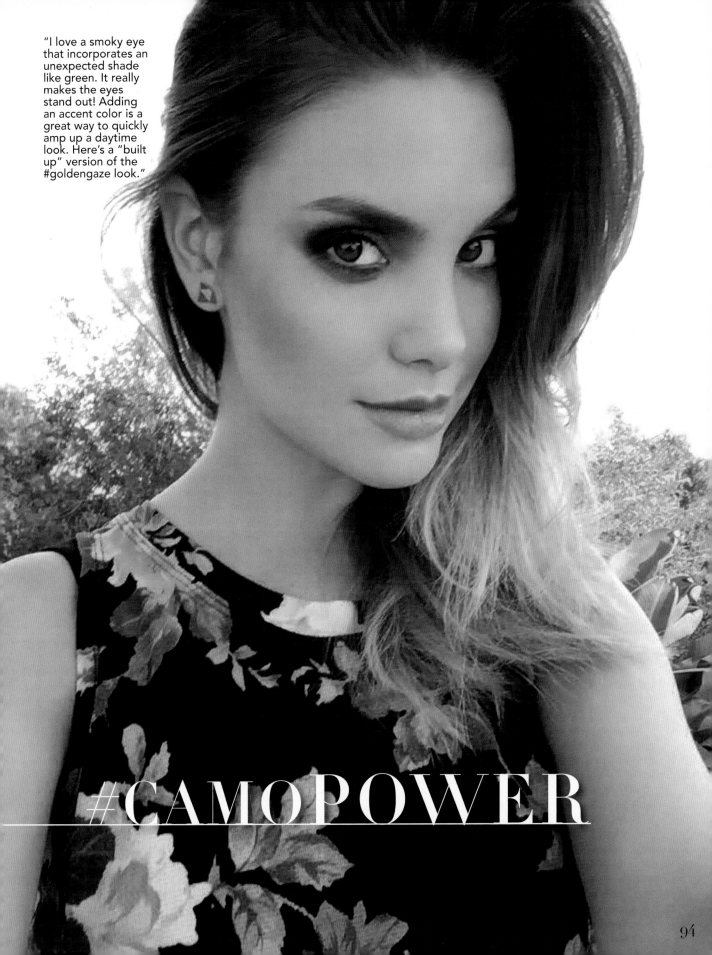

"I love a smoky eye that incorporates an unexpected shade like green. It really makes the eyes stand out! Adding an accent color is a great way to quickly amp up a daytime look. Here's a "built up" version of the #goldengaze look."

#CAMOPOWER

#LETSGROOVE

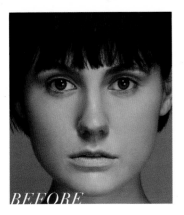

BEFORE

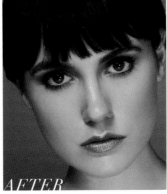

AFTER

The Essentials

- Concealer
- Blue-gray, matte gray, matte light brown and silver iridescent eyeshadows
- Eyeliner brush
- Crease brush
- Lengthening mascara
- Warm salmon cheek color
- Powder highlighter
- Velvety apricot lipstick

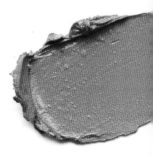

one

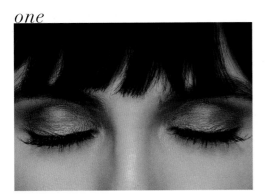

two

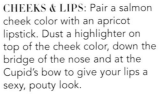

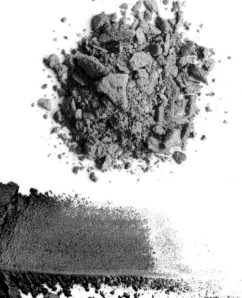

EYES: Using your concealer as a primer, apply a sheer wash all around the eyes, then tap a shimmery blue-gray eyeshadow from lash line to crease. Use an eyeliner brush to shade the entire lower lash line with a matte gray eyeshadow, then use a light brown matte shade to blend out the edges with a crease brush.

TIP: *If your eyes are small or close-set, concentrate the light brown shade on the outer three-quarters of the eyes, pulling up and out slightly at the outer corners. This will create a lifting effect on the eyes.*

EYELASHES: Curl your eyelashes. Apply a couple of coats of a lengthening mascara by holding the wand horizontally at the base of the lashes and wiggling it back and forth as you move it up.

TIP: *While the mascara is still wet, keep your eyes open, push the ends of your eyelashes up and hold for a few seconds. This is a great way to ensure that your lashes will hold their curl. Repeat with another coat on the top and bottom lashes.*

CHEEKS & LIPS: Pair a salmon cheek color with an apricot lipstick. Dust a highlighter on top of the cheek color, down the bridge of the nose and at the Cupid's bow to give your lips a sexy, pouty look.

SELFIE TIP:

Get inspired! Create your own mood board or interest board with poses and looks you'd like to try. Use them as a guide when you take your selfies!

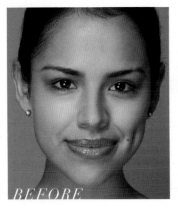

BEFORE

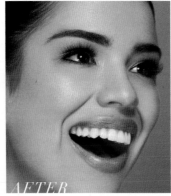

AFTER

The Essentials

- Light bone, sparkly blue and matte brown eyeshadows
- Fluffy eyeshadow brush
- Crease brush and blush brush
- Liquid highlighter
- Mascara
- Strip of false eyelashes
- Peachy copper blush and lipstick

one

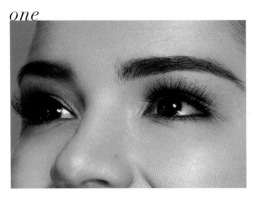

two

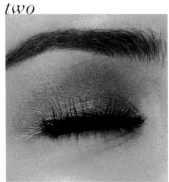

three

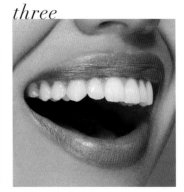

EYES: Dab an eye primer over the lid and lower lash line, then apply a light bone eyeshadow all over the lid. Next, press an iridescent blue eyeshadow along the lash line and all around the eye with an eyeliner brush. Using a fluffy eyeshadow brush, blend the blue shade and carry it up to the crease. Use the same brush to soften the lower lash line. Liberally apply a matte brown shade to the crease and blend thoroughly with a crease brush using back-and-forth windshield wiper motions.

EYELASHES: Apply one coat of mascara to the top and bottom lashes. Apply eyelash glue to the base of the fluttery faux lashes and wait until the glue becomes tacky. Use tweezers to drop the falsie strip right on top of your natural lashes, placing them as close to the base as possible. Apply another coat of mascara.

TIP: *Make sure you soften your false lashes before you apply them by bending then back and forth a few times. You may also trim them to fit.*

CHEEKS AND LIPS: Swirl a peachy copper blush right at the apples of the cheeks with a blush brush. Blend until the color disappears at the hairline. Dot a liquid highlighter onto the top of the cheeks, the bridge of the nose and any areas you'd like to illuminate. Blend well. Finish by putting on a peachy brown creamy lipstick.

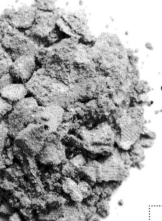

SELFIE TIP:

To create one of the most universally flattering selfie angles, hold your phone a full arm's length away from your face, about six-inches higher than your head. Tilt the phone towards you at a 45-degree angle and shoot!

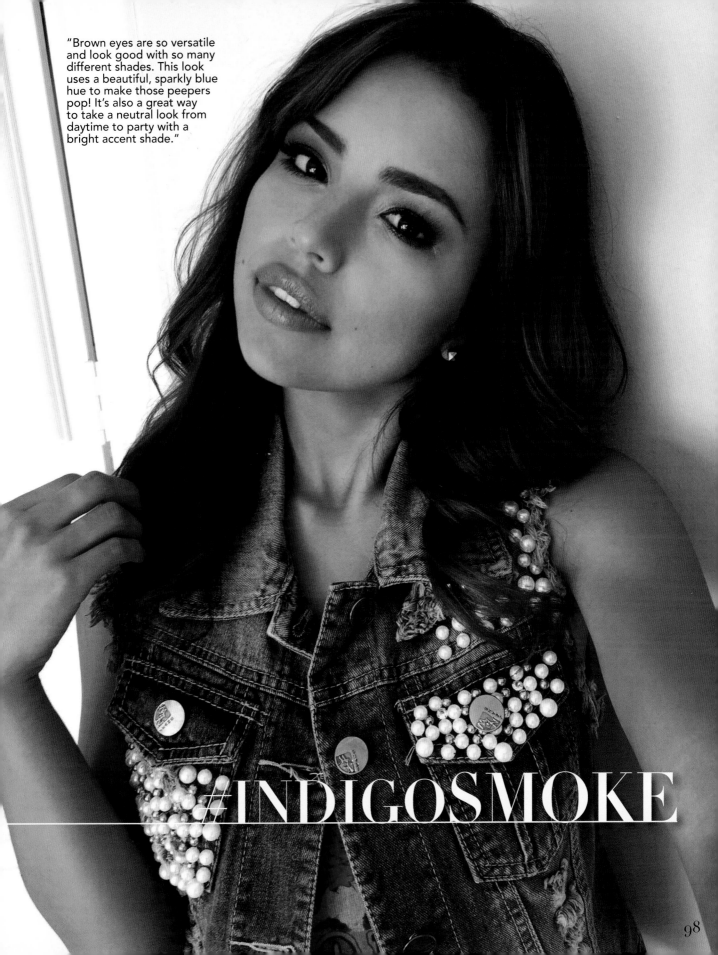

"Brown eyes are so versatile and look good with so many different shades. This look uses a beautiful, sparkly blue hue to make those peepers pop! It's also a great way to take a neutral look from daytime to party with a bright accent shade."

#INDIGoSMOKE

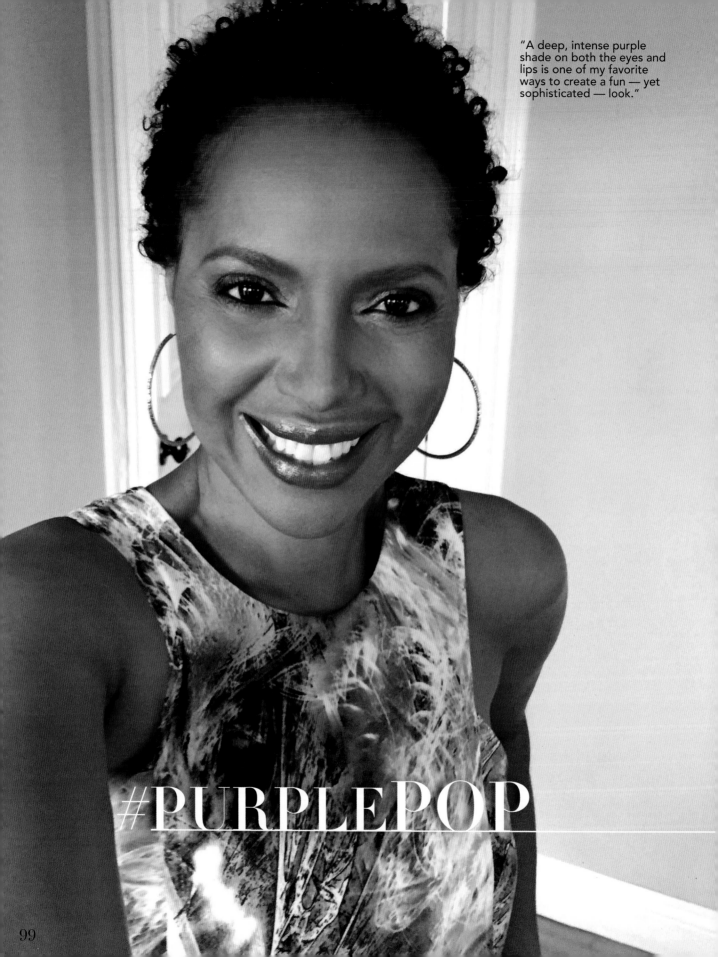

"A deep, intense purple shade on both the eyes and lips is one of my favorite ways to create a fun — yet sophisticated — look."

#PURPLEPOP

99

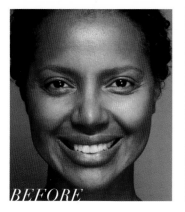

BEFORE

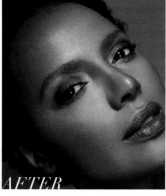

AFTER

The Essentials

- Foundation in three shades: one that matches your skin tone, one that's a shade lighter than your skin tone and one that's a shade darker than your skin tone
- Foundation brush
- Synthetic bristle eyeshadow brush
- Purple and copper eyeshadows
- Black eyeliner
- Mascara primer
- Mascara
- Golden bronze cheek color
- Rich copper-brown lipstick

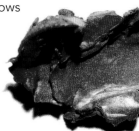

one

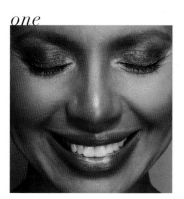

two

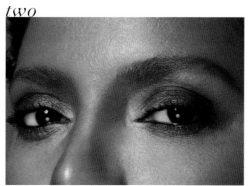

three

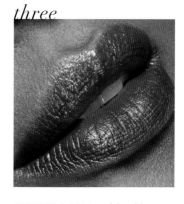

SKIN: Moisturize and prime skin, then apply a sheer wash of foundation in a shade that matches your skin tone. Using a foundation one shade lighter than your skin tone, highlight the bridge of the nose, the tops of the cheekbones and any areas you'd like to accentuate. Using a foundation one shade darker than your skin tone, contour your hairline, the sides of your nose and underneath the cheekbones. Use a sponge or a clean brush to blend all three shades together. Finish by dusting a light veil of loose powder all over the face.

TIP: *A damp blending sponge will help sheer out foundation that's too heavy.*

EYES: Apply eye primer, let dry, then use a small synthetic brush to add a sheer bronze eyeshadow to the inner corners of the eyes, the lid and along the inner half of the lower lash line. Blend edges with an eye brush. Using the same brush technique, apply a purple eyeshadow to the outer corners and along three-quarters of the outer portion of the lower lash line. Blend well. To intensify the look, add black eyeliner along the lower waterline. Finish the eyes with a mascara primer followed by two coats of lengthening mascara.

TIP: *A tight, synthetic bristle brush allows for super precise application.*

CHEEKS & LIPS: Add golden bronze shades to the cheeks and lips. Overall, darker complexions look beautiful in warm, rich hues.

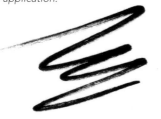

SELFIE TIP:

Watch your posture when you snap your selfie. You look amazing, so straighten your back and you hold your head up high!

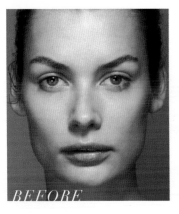

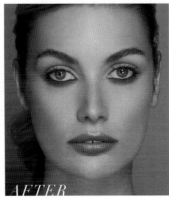

BEFORE

AFTER

The Essentials

- Concealer
- Brown, light tan and black eyeshadows
- Concealer brush
- Eyeshadow brush
- Black eyeliner
- Mascara
- Golden pink blush
- Warm pink lipstick

one

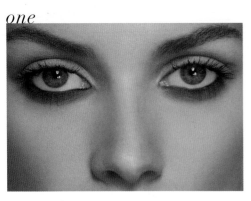

two

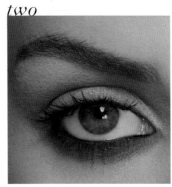

three

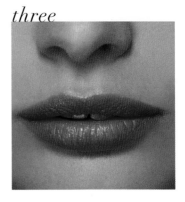

CONCEAL & PRIME: After applying foundation, prep your eyes with primer along the lower lash line and on the lid. Use a concealer brush or your ring finger to blend.

TIP: If you have dark discoloration on your lid or under your eyes, pat on a few dots of concealer and blend from the inner corners out.

EYES: Start by sweeping a matte eyeshadow that's about one shade lighter than your skin tone over the entire eyelid. Follow by applying a light brown or tan matte eyeshadow from lash line to crease and along the lower lash line. Blend the colors thoroughly. Line the lower lashes with black eyeliner, staying as close to the base of the lashes as possible. Smudge with a brush. Blend the light brown shade to create a smoky effect. Finish by applying a couple of coats of mascara to the top and bottom eyelashes.

CHEEKS AND LIPS: Apply a golden pink blush to the cheeks. Fill the lips with neutral lip liner and follow with a swipe of a warm pink lipstick.

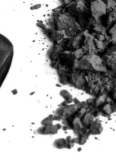

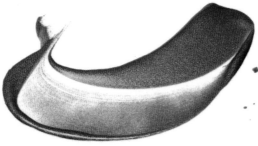

SELFIE TIP:

When sporting a heavy eyeliner look, make sure to take your selfie in soft, natural light. It will make your skin look soft and glowy and will nicely illuminate your face.

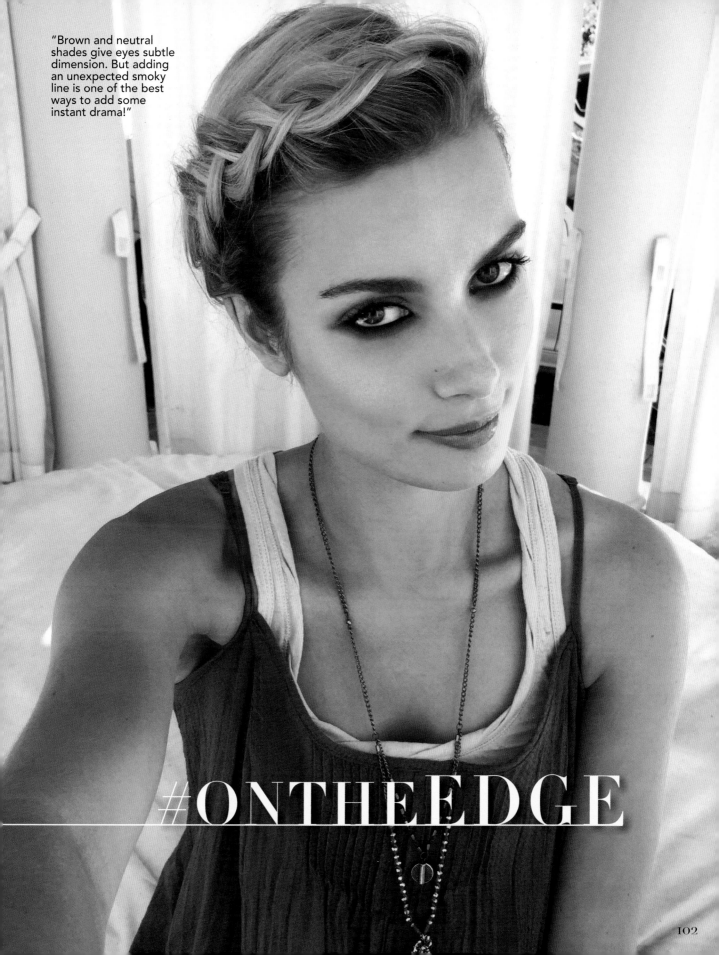

"Brown and neutral shades give eyes subtle dimension. But adding an unexpected smoky line is one of the best ways to add some instant drama!"

#ONtheEDGE

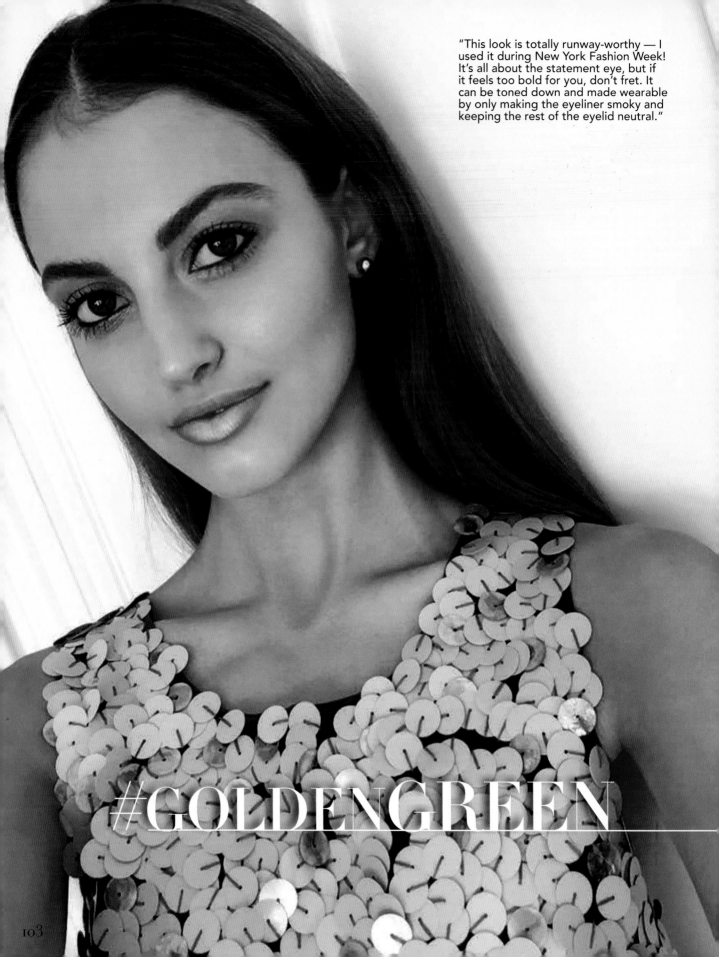

"This look is totally runway-worthy — I used it during New York Fashion Week! It's all about the statement eye, but if it feels too bold for you, don't fret. It can be toned down and made wearable by only making the eyeliner smoky and keeping the rest of the eyelid neutral."

#GOLDENGREEN

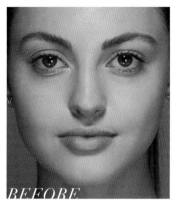

BEFORE

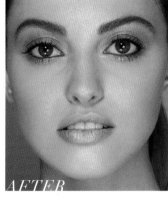

AFTER

The Essentials

- Foundation
- Translucent powder
- Gold, emerald-green and soft aqua-blue eye-shadows
- Black gel or liquid eyeliner
- Mascara
- Warm brown-gold cheek color
- Sheer nude iridescent lipstick

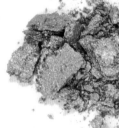

one

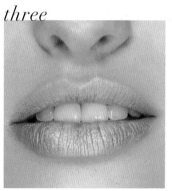

two

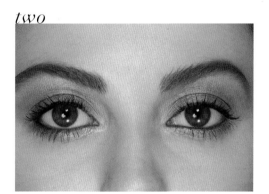

three

SKIN: Starting at the nose, apply a light, sheer foundation and blend downward with a brush. Continue blending until the foundation disappears at the hair and jawlines. Apply a second layer of foundation across the forehead and blend, concentrating on the areas that need extra coverage. Set with a light dusting of powder.

EYES: Apply an eye primer or a light green crayon all over the eyelid, carrying it underneath the lower lash line. Tap warm gold eyeshadow in the inner corners of the eye, on the lid and under the lower lash line. Layer an emerald-green shade over the gold and carry it slightly above your crease. Finish by applying a light blue eyeshadow to the crease and blend any edges away. Use a very thin swipe of black gel eyeliner, then apply two coats of mascara on the top and lower lashes.

CHEEKS & LIPS: Use a blush one shade darker than your skin tone to sculpt the cheeks (remember not to add any more color to the look). Apply a light, nude lipstick with a hint of sparkle to the lips.

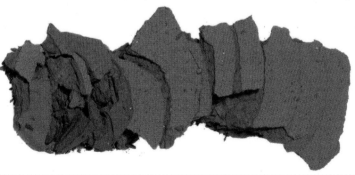

SELFIE TIP:

Use your camera's best resolution. Go to your smartphone's settings and make sure you use the highest resolution available. And yes, delete any unwanted photos on a regular basis to avoid overloading your phone's memory.

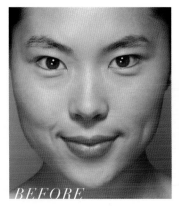

BEFORE

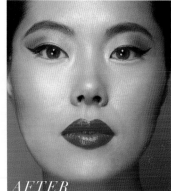

AFTER

The Essentials

- Matte foundation one shade darker than your skin tone
- Luminous liquid foundation that matches your skin tone
- Translucent powder
- Concealer
- Highlighter
- Taupe and copper eyeshadows
- Gel or liquid eyeliner
- Mascara
- Golden pink blush
- Red lipstick and lip gloss

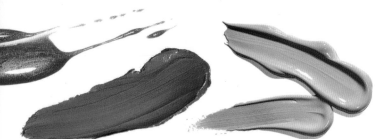

one

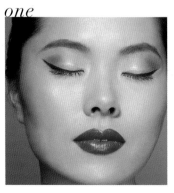

two

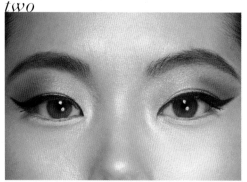

three

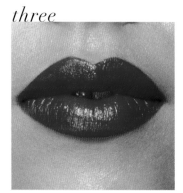

SKIN: Moisturize and prime the skin, giving each product ample time to dry. Using a matte foundation one shade darker than your skin tone, contour the hollows of the cheeks with a foundation brush. Use what's left on your brush to sculpt the temples and the jawline. Follow by applying a luminous finish foundation that matches your skin to the center of the face. Use a damp sponge to blend, then apply with concealer where needed. Finish with a light dusting of translucent powder.

EYES: Pat a light taupe eyeshadow from the lash line up, allowing the color to fade under the brows. Starting at the outer corner of the eyes, apply a warm copper eyeshadow with an eyeshadow brush and blend until the color creates a soft shadow along the outer third of the eye and the crease. Dust the light taupe eyeshadow along the lower lash line to brighten up the eyes.

TIP: *This is a great technique for hooded or monolid eyes!*

EYELINER: Use a gel or liquid eyeliner to draw a line from the inner corner out. Thicken the line as you move towards the outer corner and flick it up at the end. Finish with a coat of mascara.

TIP: *If you're nervous about using liquid eyeliner, use a black eyeliner pencil to create your winged shape, then trace over the shape with liquid liner.*

CHEEKS AND LIPS: Exfoliate and moisturize your lips while you make up the rest of the face. Swipe a red lipstick right on to the lips and use a lip brush to perfect the shape. Blot and reapply. Add a drop of bright red lip gloss to the center of the lips. Finish the look with a golden pink blush.

TIP: *Perfect your lip shape by applying a bit of foundation with a brush around the lip line.*

SELFIE TIP:

It pays to be precise when wearing a strong lip look in your selfie! Whether you're using a lip brush or applying lipstick straight from the tube, be mindful of outlining your lips — wonky lines will show!

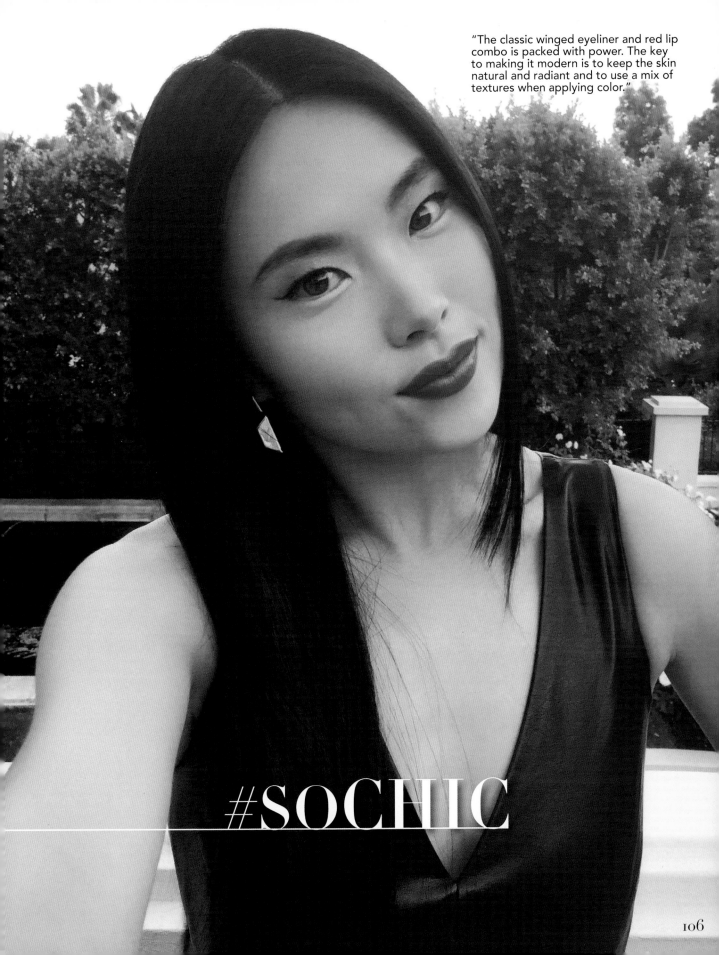

"The classic winged eyeliner and red lip combo is packed with power. The key to making it modern is to keep the skin natural and radiant and to use a mix of textures when applying color."

#SOCHIC

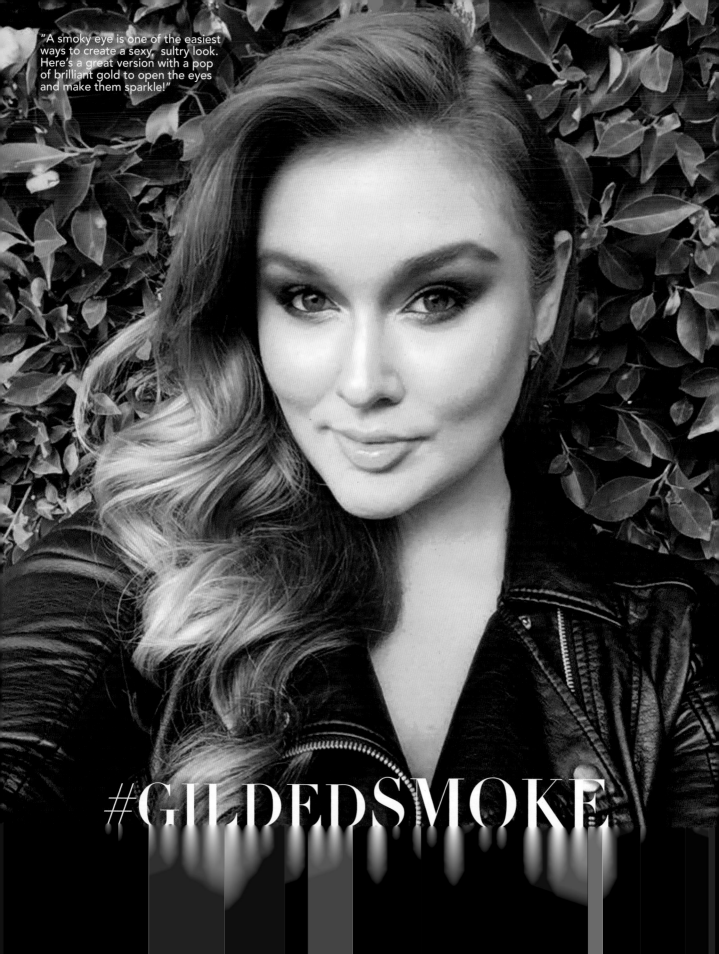

"A smoky eye is one of the easiest ways to create a sexy, sultry look. Here's a great version with a pop of brilliant gold to open the eyes and make them sparkle!"

#GILDEDSMOKE

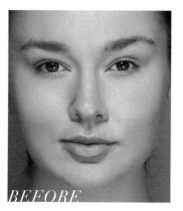
BEFORE

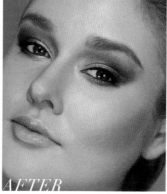
AFTER

The Essentials

- Bone, pink-brown, gold and dark charcoal eye-shadows
- Black pencil or gel eyeliner
- Mascara
- Bronzer
- Warm pink cheek color
- Neutral lip liner
- Nude lipstick

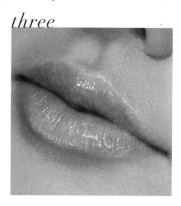

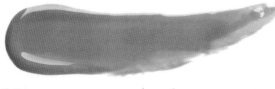

one

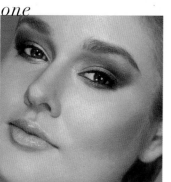

two

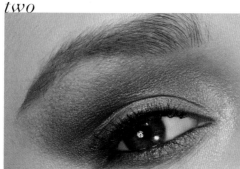

three

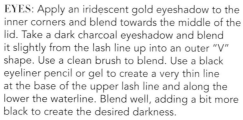

PREP & PRIME: Pat an eye primer onto the lids and up to the brows. Even out any skin discoloration by applying concealer to the inner corners and underneath the eyes.

EYES: Apply an iridescent gold eyeshadow to the inner corners and blend towards the middle of the lid. Take a dark charcoal eyeshadow and blend it slightly from the lash line up into an outer "V" shape. Use a clean brush to blend. Use a black eyeliner pencil or gel to create a very thin line at the base of the upper lash line and along the lower the waterline. Blend well, adding a bit more black to create the desired darkness.

EYELASHES: Curl lashes and follow with a coat of regular mascara. Apply a coat of waterproof mascara to both the upper and lower lashes for maximum, long-lasting impact.

CHEEKS & LIPS: Using a cheek brush, dust a warm pink cheek color onto the hollows of the cheeks. Blend from the tops of the cheeks to the temples with a clean brush. Fill the lips with a neutral lip liner and finish with a nude lipstick.

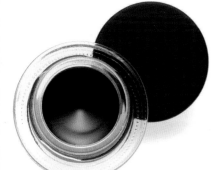

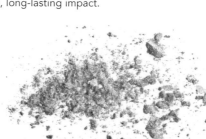

SELFIE TIP:
When wearing a stand-out makeup look, keep your background simple. When in doubt, position yourself in front of a plain wall or simple backdrop.

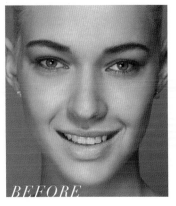
BEFORE

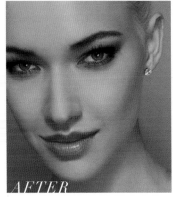
AFTER

The Essentials

- Translucent powder
- Liquid highlighter
- Deep blue, black and silver-gray eye-shadows
- Eyeliner or smudge brushes
- Waterproof mascara
- Golden bronze cheek color
- Sheer nude lipstick

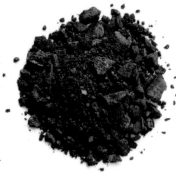

one

two

three

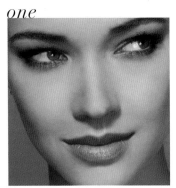
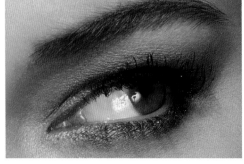
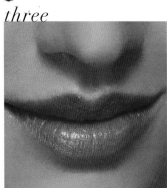

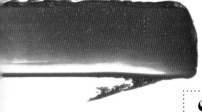

SKIN: To freshen up the look and illuminate the face, apply a few dots of liquid highlighter to the upper cheeks, forehead, inner eye corners and brow bone. Follow with translucent powder where needed.

EYES: With an eyeshadow brush, intensify the silver-gray eyeshadow by sweeping another layer across the upper lid to the crease, under the lower lashes and into the inner corners. Use a smudge brush to press a bright blue eye color along the lower lash line. Blend to soften. Heighten the smoky effect by blending the coal black eyeshadow along the upper lash line, then out onto the outer third of the eyelid. Finish with another coat of waterproof mascara.

TIP: *When you are finished applying eyeshadow, apply concealer in a "V" shape to the under-eye area. Blend up until it disappears completely.*

CHEEKS AND LIPS: Add a warmer cheek color to the hollows of the cheeks and blend into the original blush. Finish the look with a sheer nude lipstick, applying it straight from the tube. Blot and reapply.

SELFIE TIP:
When taking your selfie with a phone, try removing the case when using the front camera. You'll be surprised how much clearer the pictures will look!

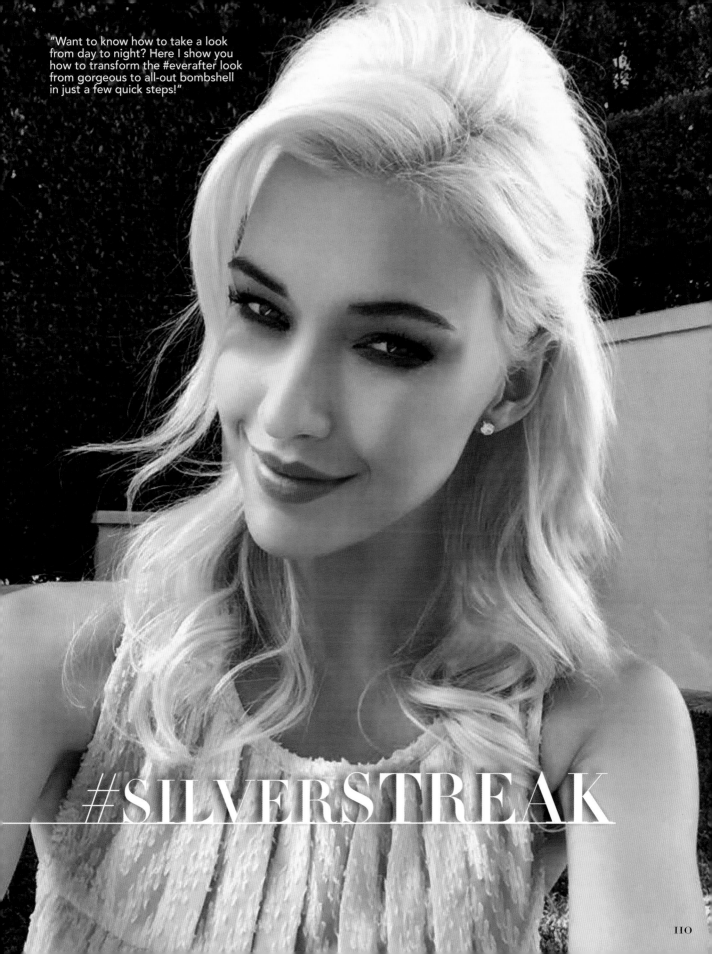

"Want to know how to take a look from day to night? Here I show you how to transform the #everafter look from gorgeous to all-out bombshell in just a few quick steps!"

#SILVERSTREAK

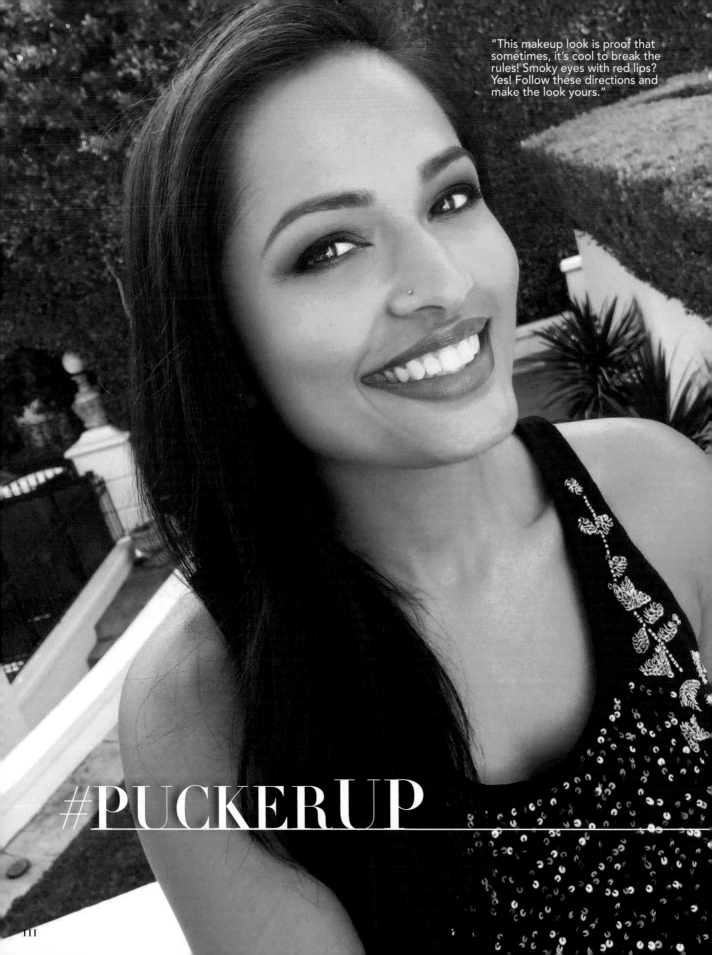

"This makeup look is proof that sometimes, it's cool to break the rules! Smoky eyes with red lips? Yes! Follow these directions and make the look yours."

#PUCKERUP

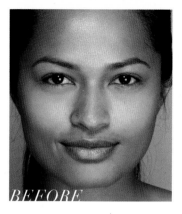
BEFORE

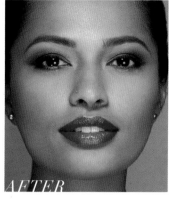
AFTER

The Essentials

- Neutral matte eyeshadows in gold-beige, brown and charcoal
- Angled eyeliner brush
- Mascara
- Lip exfoliator and moisturizer
- Warm peach blush
- Creamy red lipstick
- Neutral lip liner the same color as your lips
- Red lip gloss

one

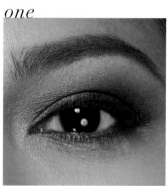

two

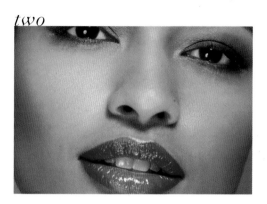

three

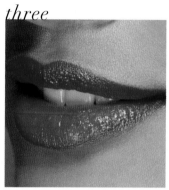

EYES: Apply a sparkly gold-beige eyeshadow to the lid. Sweep a matte brown eyeshadow on top and into the crease. Carry the shadow along the bottom lash line, working from the outer corner in. To create the smoky look, layer a charcoal-black eyeshadow over the outer third of the upper eyelid and along three-quarters of the lower lash line. Blend, then rim the top lash line with a black eyeshadow using an angled brush. Extend the line past the outer corner to make the eye appear larger. Curl your lashes and add mascara to both top and bottom.

TIP: *Afraid of smudges while creating your smoky eye? Try using a business card as a shield. Align the card with your lower lash line and hold it in place while you blend the eyeshadows together. You can also use a piece of tape.*

CHEEKS: Dust a warm peach blush along the hollows of the cheeks. Blend the blush up to the apples of the cheeks, then in a "C" shape along the sides of your face up to your temples. Apply highlighter to the center of the nose, the Cupid's bow and the brow bone.

TIP: *You can find the hollows of your cheeks by making a "fish face" in front of the mirror. The sunken in area is where you want to apply your blush.*

LIPS: Start by exfoliating and moisturizing the lips to ensure a smooth, long-lasting application. Smooth on a very light amount of foundation to neutralize any discoloration. Apply red, creamy lipstick straight from the tube onto the bottom lip and blot. Repeat if needed. With a lip liner that matches the shade of your lips, start at the Cupid's bow and carry the color to the outer corners for a precise look. If necessary, apply a sheer red gloss on top.

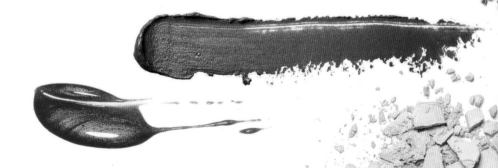

SELFIE TIP:

Get to know your smartphone camera! Experimenting with its resolution, filters and other unique functions will give you the best results. There are so many things a smartphone can do with photos!

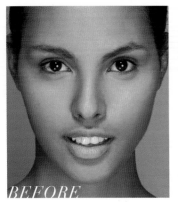

BEFORE

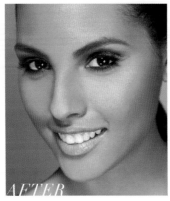

AFTER

The Essentials

- Gold cream eyeshadow
- Copper, black and gold eyeshadows
- Black eyeliner
- Mascara primer
- Mascara
- Cheek color one shade darker than your skin tone
- Nude lip gloss

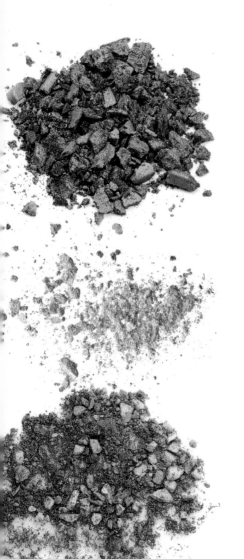

one

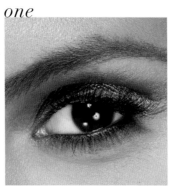

EYES: Use a gold cream eyeshadow as a base all around the eye, then tap a copper shade onto the lid and the lower lash line with a tight synthetic eyeshadow brush. Blend with a clean brush at the crease and soften the lower lash line. Finish with a tight line of black eyeshadow along the lower lash line and soften it slightly into the copper shade.

two

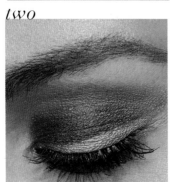

EYELINER: With an angled brush, apply a line of gold cream eyeshadow to the base of the upper lashes. Start at the inner corners and widen the line slightly as you move towards the outer corners. Swipe a bright gold eyeshadow on top and repeat if necessary.

TIP: *Iridescent eyeshadows work best for this technique because they dry to a beautiful sheen.*

EYELASHES: Use a mascara primer before applying a couple of coats of mascara.

TIP: *Black mascara neutralizes a bright eyeliner, so make sure to play up your lashes!*

three

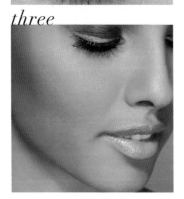

CHEEKS & LIPS: A look like this calls for a cheek color that's about one shade darker than your skin tone. Finish with a iridescent nude lip gloss.

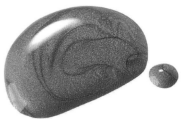

SELFIE TIP:

Don't use the same filter for all your selfies! Even though there are some great ones that seem to work perfectly with every shot, I recommend trying a variety after you've taken your selfies. One size doesn't fit all, and switching up your filters can give you fantastic results.

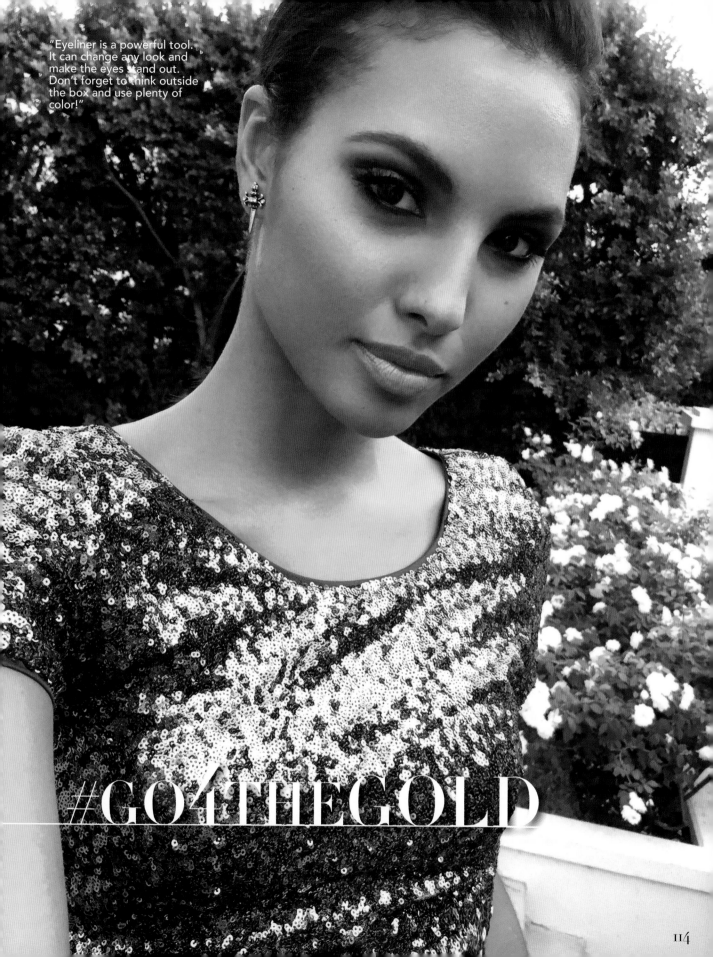

"Eyeliner is a powerful tool. It can change any look and make the eyes stand out. Don't forget to think outside the box and use plenty of color!"

#GO4THEGOLD

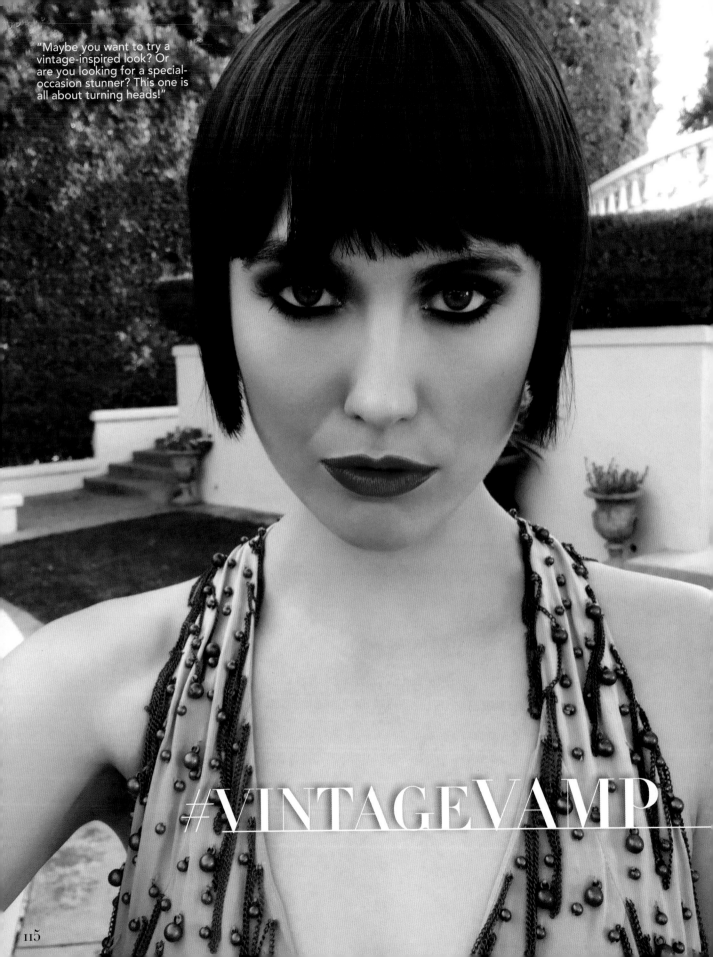

"Maybe you want to try a vintage-inspired look? Or are you looking for a special-occasion stunner? This one is all about turning heads!"

#VINTAGEVAMP

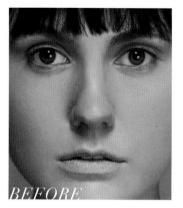
BEFORE

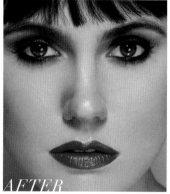
AFTER

The Essentials

- Matte finish foundation
- Concealer
- Liquid highlighter
- Silver and black eyeshadows
- Flat eyeshadow brush
- Eyeliner brush
- Black eyeliner
- Mascara
- Bronzer
- Coral cheek color
- Red and orange-red lipstick
- Neutral lip liner

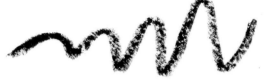

one

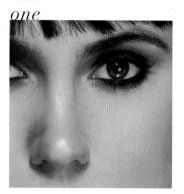

two

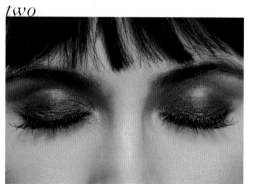

three

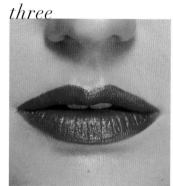

SKIN: Moisturize and prime. Apply a matte finish foundation sparingly and in layers where extra coverage is needed. Wait until you've finished making up your eyes, then use concealer where necessary and create a "V" shape under the eyes with a liquid highlighter. Blend well.

EYES: Apply eye primer, which is a must when wearing bold eye makeup. With a flat brush, tap a silver eyeshadow onto the lid from the top lash line to the crease and along the lower lash line, concentrating on the inner corners. Use an eyeliner brush to tap a coal-black eyeshadow right at the lash line all around the eye. Blend with a clean eyeshadow brush to create a smoky effect. Finish by tracing a thin line of black eyeliner along the waterline or at the base of the lower lashes. Curl lashes and apply two coats of mascara on the top and bottom.

CHEEKS & LIPS: Sculpt the face with a bronzer. Follow with a coral cheek color that's blended with the bronzer for a soft warming effect. Add highlighter if desired. Exfoliate and moisturize lips, then apply a creamy orange-red lipstick straight from the tube. Layer with a darker red lipstick for a modern ombré effect. Line the lips to perfect their shape, blot and repeat.

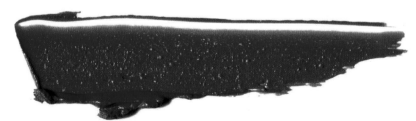

SELFIE TIP:
Capture this 1920s look with a cool vintage filter in black and white!

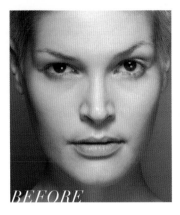

BEFORE

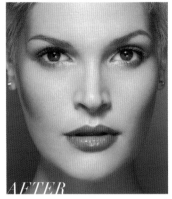

AFTER

The Essentials

- Translucent powder
- Sparkly white, light beige, copper-brown, pink-brown and matte or soft shimmery nude-beige eyeshadows
- Brown or black eyeliner
- Waterproof mascara
- Bronzy pink cheek color
- Red lipstick

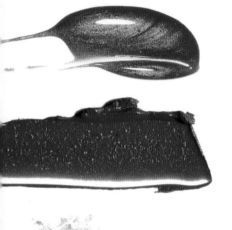

one

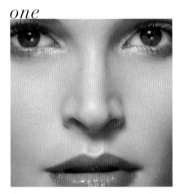

SKIN: Start by moisturizing your face and using an eye cream. Follow with a face primer and a radiant, luminous foundation. Give your face a youthful lift by applying a golden pink blush right at the apple of your cheeks. Set with translucent powder.

TIP: *You can add a tiny bit of liquid highlighter to the tops of your cheekbones and onto your brow bone to reflect and lift the whole face.*

two

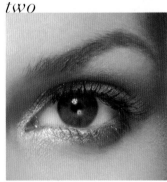

EYES: Apply a light beige eyeshadow all over the eye area. Define the crease and shade two thirds of the lower lash line with a copper brown eyeshadow. Blend out the edges with a pink-brown eyeshadow. Apply brown or black eyeliner at the lash line and brighten the inner corners of the eyes with a sparkly white eyeshadow.

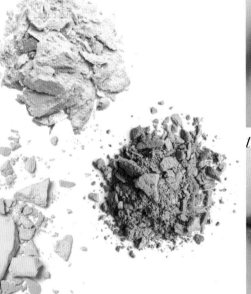

three

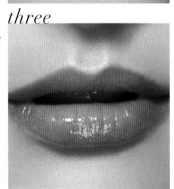

LIPS: Over lip balm, apply a tiny bit of foundation to neutralize any undertones on your lips. Line the lips with a neutral or nude lip liner if necessary. Then pick a shade of red lipstick according to your skin type:

Fair skin: Corals and soft red

Medium skin: True red and light berry tones

Dark skin: Burgundy or brick

SELFIE TIP:

Matte or glossy? It's your choice. Matte is a classic look, while glossy will add a youthful shine!

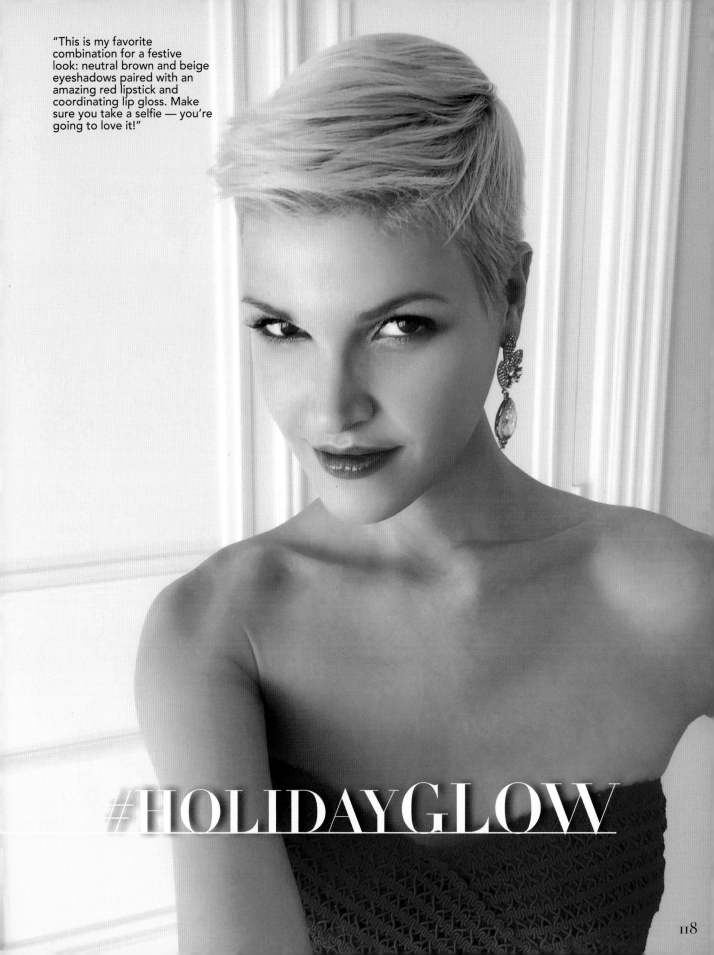

"This is my favorite combination for a festive look: neutral brown and beige eyeshadows paired with an amazing red lipstick and coordinating lip gloss. Make sure you take a selfie — you're going to love it!"

#HOLIDAYGLOW

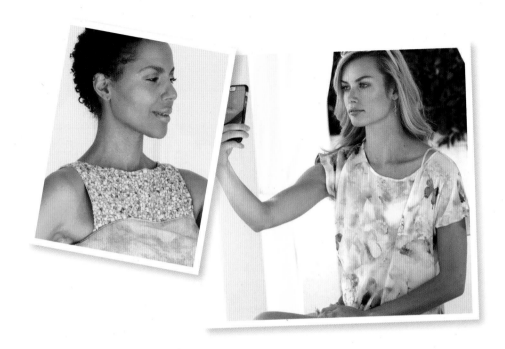

Behind the Scenes

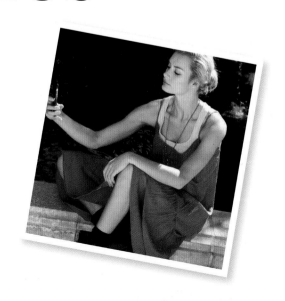

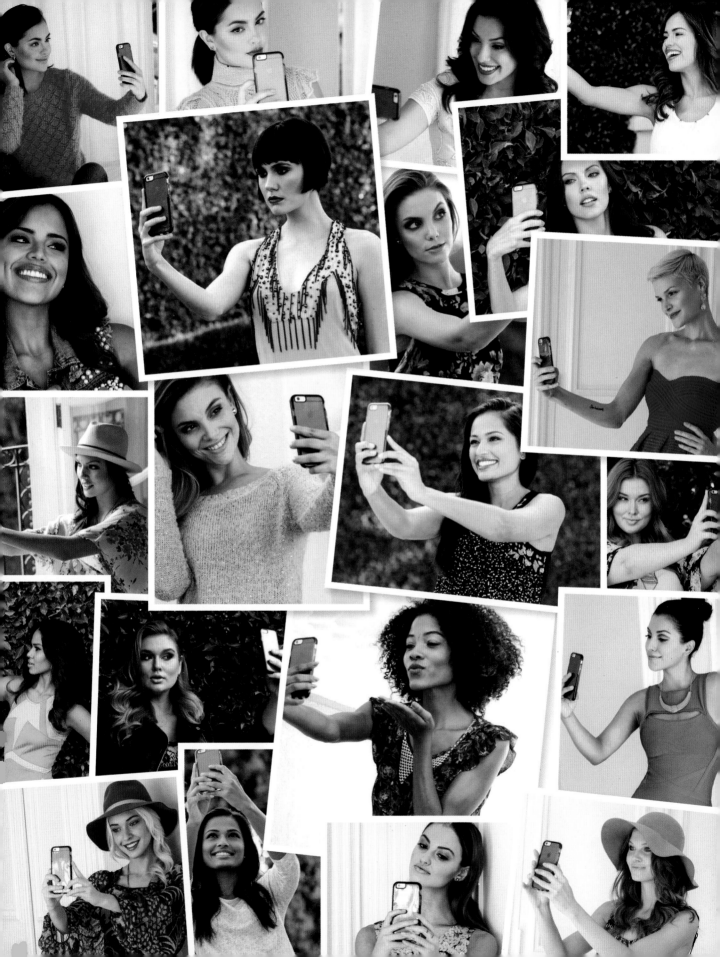

Special Thanks

I couldn't have finished this project without these amazing people:

Sheryl Adkins-Green • Peter Augustin • Jeanna Bonello • Andy Bonura • Ryan Burchfield
CloutierRemix • Birgit Dhonau • Amanda Van Duyse • Ciara Gay • Paul Jones • Gwen Kellet
Nancy Lan • Madeline Leonard • Jenny Laible • Susan Linney • Justin Loy • Molly Magill
Brett McCall • Matty Miyamoto • MML PR • Sylvia Molina • Abigail Nieto • Daniel Palacios
Judy Pham • Marianny Rojas • Barbara Sagami • Eva Sarakay • Kim Sater • Frank Sebastian
Jennifer Shaffer • David Sorafine • Veronica Soto • Virginia Soto • Kori Stanton
Shannon Summers • Emma Trask • Josh Williams
and a special thanks to Stephen Webster

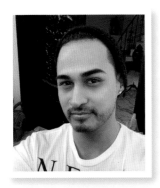
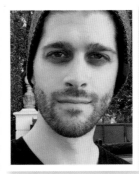
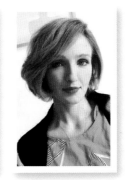
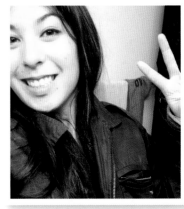

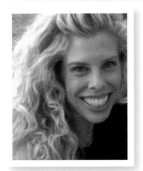
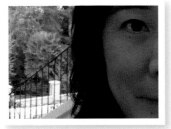
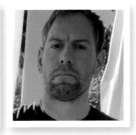
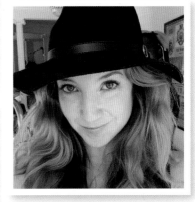

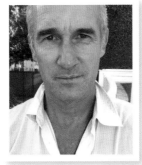
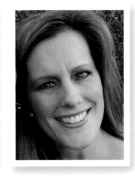

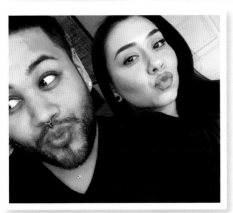
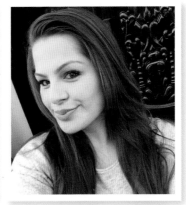
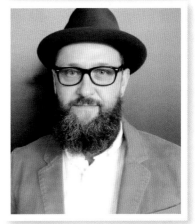

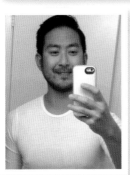
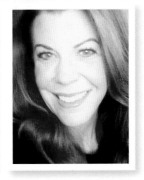
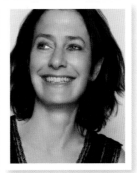
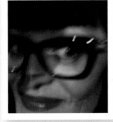

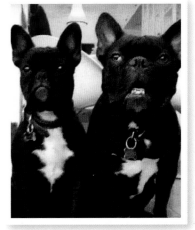

Index